IMAGES OF HEALING

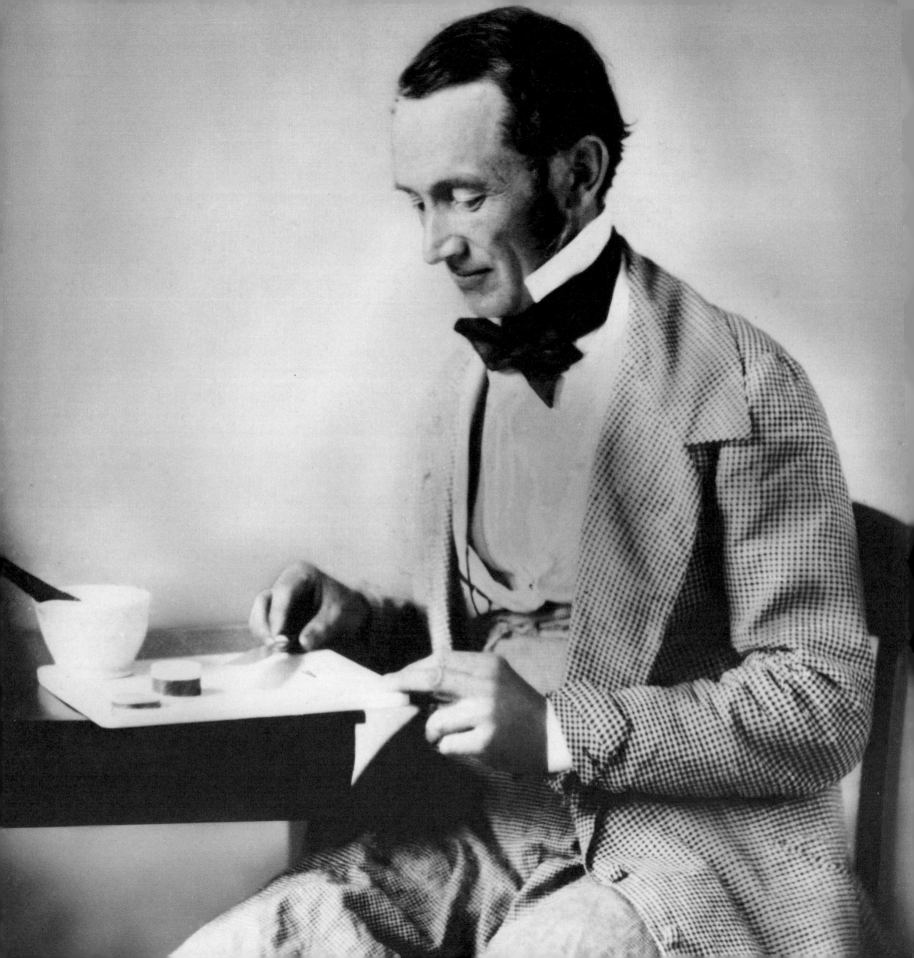

IMAGES OF HEALING

A Portfolio of American Medical & Pharmaceutical Practice in the 18th, 19th, & early 20th Centuries

Edited by Ann Novotny & Carter Smith with an introduction by William D. Sharpe, M.D.

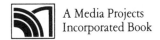

A Media Projects
Incorporated Book

MACMILLAN PUBLISHING CO., INC., New York
COLLIER MACMILLAN PUBLISHERS, London

Title page photograph: Henry Brewer, of the
H. & J. Brewer Drugstore, Springfield, Mass.
Daguerreotype, c. 1850. [M.1.]

Macmillan Publishing Co., Inc.
866 Third Avenue, New York, New York 10022
Collier Macmillan Canada, Ltd.

Library of Congress Cataloging in Publication Data
Main entry under title:

Images of healing.

1. Medicine—United States—History—Pictorial works.
2. Pharmacy—United States—History—Pictorial works.
I. Novotny, Ann. II. Smith, Carter, 1931-
[DNLM: 1. History of medicine, 18th century—United States. 2. History of
medicine, 19th century—United States. 3. History of medicine, 20th
century—United States. 4. History of dentistry—United States. 5. Pharmacy—History—United States. WZ70 AA1 I3]
R151.I49   610'.973   80-15701
ISBN 0-02-590820-0

Images of Healing was created by Media Projects Incorporated in association
with Prose & Concepts, Inc.

Project Staff:
  Editor: Carter Smith
  Consulting Editors: Ann Novotny and William D. Sharpe, M.D.
  Project Editor: Beverly Gary Kempton
  Assistant Editors: Ellen Coffey and Alix Gudefin Perrachon
  Researchers: Linda Christenson, Sarah Goodyear, and Jacqueline Polin
  Dust jacket and book design: Bryan Dew
  Assistant Designer / Production Supervisor: Derek Dalton
  Production Assistant: Claude D. Doswell

10   9   8   7   6   5   4   3   2   1

Printed in the United States of America

Contents

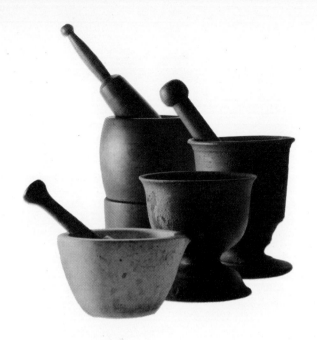

Foreword

When humans came to inherit the earth, they found themselves burdened with a bewildering array of diseases. So formidable was this threat to life one must marvel at the ability of *Homo sapiens* to hold their supremacy. Prehistoric art indicates that man even then had achieved mastery over the most ferocious animals, but he has long been frustrated by his inability to win biological dominance in the world of microorganisms. And microorganisms are the cause of many of his diseases.

During the Renaissance, a time of enormous commercial expansion, explorers and adventurers brought as much zeal to their quest for healing substances as to the search for precious metals. Indeed, the "magic potions" of the New World vastly enriched the European materia medica.

In 1607, after King James I granted the London Company a charter to all the territory between the Spanish settlements in Florida and the French ones in Canada, two "apothycaries" accompanied the first English colonists to debark at Hampton Roads. In later correspondence to London, the Virginia Company urgently requested, "some Phisitians and Apothycaries of which we stand much need of."

Above: Antique Mortars and Pestles. [H.M.S]. *Front to rear:* stone (pestle handle, wood); brass mortar, pestle missing; iron mortar and pestle, hand cast; wood mortar and pestle. Today most are glass or ceramic and pharmacists are required by law to have such equipment.

Neither physicians nor pharmacists, however, flocked to the American colonies. Much like other young societies, health care in the colonies was largely administered by housewives, who concocted remedies from indigenous herbs with medicinal properties. The colonists also had access to a host of packaged secret nostrums, "legalized" by the British Parliament in 1624. Many were there who set forth to face the hazards of the New World equipped with a box of Anderson's Scot Pills, or a bottle of Daffy's Elixir Salutis. To the busy settler with scant time and means, these comparatively inexpensive remedies, with their extravagant claims, were of obvious appeal.

The status of medical knowledge at the beginning of the 18th century permitted patent medicines to find a comfortable niche in the environment, for men knew little more about the origins of diseases than had the ancient Greeks. Then too, the aristocratic practitioners of the London College of Physicians were few in number and closed in rank. The masses had to seek care elsewhere, and turned to the apothecaries (who obtained a special status as minor practitioners by a 1617 act of King James I), the surgeons (more often than not members of the Barbers' Guild), the chemists and druggists (the wholesale and retail merchants of crude drugs), and the entrepreneurs of the "patented" quack remedies.

In colonial America, the lines were drawn even less sharply. A New Englander in 1690 observed that, "surgeons & midwives are dignified acc(ording) to successe."

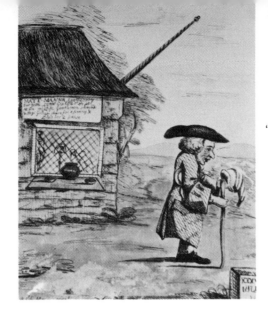

Matthea Manna, The Country Apothecary. 18th century engraving by R. St. G. Mansergh. [P.C.] The shop sign reads: "Apothecary, Surgeon, Corn Cutter, Etc., Etc., Man midwife . . ."

Drug Mill. Engraving, late 19th century. [P.C.] Maker: H. Troemner, Phila.; Patented, January 17, 1870.

One of the first pharmacies in the colonies was established not by an Englishman or Scotsman, but by the Dutch surgeon Gysbert van Imbroch, who "kept a shop at New Amsterdam" in 1653. The earliest known account book of a practising pharmacist—commencing in 1698—belonged to Bartholowmew Browne of Salem, Massachusetts. It is significant that he described himself as a "pharmaceutical chemist" rather than an apothecary, the first evidence that a new profession was emerging.

By 1730, when this Portfolio of American Medical & Pharmaceutical Practice begins, the foundations were established. In 1721, despite violent opposition, American-born medical practitioner Zabdiel Boylston of Boston had inoculated his only son for smallpox; and about 1726, Elizabeth Greenleaf (preceding by nearly a century Elizabeth Marshall, who is so often cited as the first woman to practice pharmacy in America) had founded the Boston-based Greenleaf Apothecary Shop. Another pioneer pharmaceutical enterprise was founded in Philadelphia in 1729 by Irish immigrant Christopher Marshall. Not only did these shops provide sorely needed medical supplies to the Continental Army and Navy during the Revolutionary War, but later, Marshall's shop was to serve as the springboard for America's first College of Pharmacy.

In 1778, Apothecary General Andrew Craigie initiated the large-scale manufacturing of drugs for the Continental Army, and immediately after the Revolutionary War, the Marshalls of Philadelphia launched an American pharmaceutical industry. The founding of the U.S. Pharmacopoeia in 1820 was a major step in the development of American medical care, as was the founding of the American Medical Association in 1847. Five years later a handful of "pharmaceutists and druggists" met in Philadelphia and established the American Pharmaceutical Association to curb traffic in adulterated drugs and poisons, investigate secret medicines and quackery, and set educational standards. With the formation of the American Dental Association in 1859, and the American Nurses Association in 1896, the organizational structure of the major segments of the health care team was complete.

As you scan this unique collection of illustrations, do not be dismayed by the evidence of man's gullibility. But neither be complacent about the impressive advances made during the two centuries covered. Rather, think upon Louis Lasanga's prophecy in *The Doctor's Dilemma:*

"In the beginning, there was Ignorance. And in the end, also, one can safely prophesy, when the last radioactive cloud settles over the hills and valley of a dead world, some wise being looking down from another planet will roar with cosmic laughter at the stupid things earth people believed about their bodies and ailments."

George B. Griffenhagen, R.Ph.

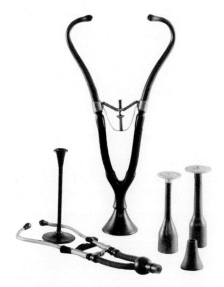

Introduction

This book is not a history of medical practice in the United States from 1730 to 1930, or of nursing, public health, pharmacy, or hospital architecture. Rather, it is an attempt to open some archives and to explore some attics. It makes no apology for being a collection of pictures that permits the reader a glimpse of the people, artifacts, documents, institutions and techniques of the healing professions during these two centuries. It hopes to place them in their social context, and as we shall see, for most people, most of the time, the good old days were actually pretty bad. Although it tries to avoid the trite, by necessity it includes much that is familiar: Pennsylvania, Massachusetts General, Bellevue and Johns Hopkins Hospitals had, and continue to have, leading roles in American medical care. Ephraim McDowell, William Beaumont, and J. Marion Sims *were* important by any standard.

American, and British North American, medical practice descended directly from that of 18th century England. Fellows of the Royal College of Physicians were occasionally capable, often learned, and usually prosperous men, but their numbers were few; most Englishmen received their medical care from surgeons and apothecaries trained by apprenticeship with only limited didactic instruction.

Above: 19th Century Stethoscopes. [H.M.S.] Three monaural stethoscopes, c. 1840. *Left:* Ebony. *Right:* Fruitwood. *Center:* Two binaural stethoscopes, c. 1860. The two ear-type instruments were an 1850 modification of René Théophile Hyacinthe Laennec's 1825 invention.

A lad finished his common schooling at 16 or 17, and was apprenticed. University degrees and examining boards were simply irrelevant until the second quarter of the 19th century, and many people knew and practiced *some* medicine. For the past century, the law has been fairly clear as to who may and may not represent himself as a medical practitioner, but with the rise of physicians' assistants, nurse practitioners, and various cults, the lines are again blurring. By custom, the 18th century physician was paid for his advice and did not dispense drugs, while the surgeons and apothecaries gave free advice and charged for drugs and surgical procedures. So began the American tradition that a doctor has not really earned a fee if he does not *give* something or *do* something. These surgeons and apothecaries were numerous, their formal qualifications vague, and their incomes modest.

Physicians, in the 18th century British sense, did not emigrate to the United States, but apothecaries did, and brought with them the tradition of apprenticeship, and therapeutic activism. Thus was general medical practice in the British fashion recreated in the colonies. The small population of the colonies, however, meant that most physicians could not support themselves by full-time practice, and until the demands of the Second World War, the typical American general practitioner often supplemented his fees with non-medical, part-time work.

The early American medical schools assumed students had served several years as apprentices, and hence taught medicine by lecture, with only sporadic demonstrations in chemistry, and superficial anatomic dissection. The graduates proved superior to the system, and despite talk about the inadequacies of American medical education before the Flexner era, there is little evidence to support the notion that practitioners in the United States were less qualified than those elsewhere. The medical schools may have been jokes, but the doctors were not.

Initially, little in the medical profession had its beginnings in America. Except for those French-speaking physicians in Louisiana and Quebec, who looked to Paris, American medicine had its roots in England. Surviving libraries and probate inventories suggest the steady importation of English books and journals; later English material was frequently reprinted in the United States for local use. And as individual interests, time, and financial resources permitted, the earliest American students went to England and Scotland for clinical training.

America's first cities—Boston, New York, New Orleans, and in particular Philadelphia—were not only hubs for shipping and commerce, but medical centers as well. However, the majority of Americans lived on farms and in small villages, and as they moved West or to the new South, their physicians and pharmacists did the same. It is customary for historians of social medicine, with scant knowledge of medical practice, to mock the twelve-bed hospital in a private dwelling, and proprietary medical schools above grocery stores. But hospital beds were needed, and doctors had to be trained. That some of these foundations were not good is undeniable, but others were the ancestors of such distinguished medical centers as those in Chicago, St. Louis, New Orleans, Houston, and San Francisco.

Interestingly, ophthalmology was a distinct specialty by mid 19th century, and because doctors and patients take eyes very seriously and are reluctant to entrust them to amateurs, its practitioners were spared the suspicion of quackery that physicians claiming to be specialists then attracted. Apart from ophthalmology, however, American physicians generally maintained the surgeon-apothecary's tradition, and put their hands to pretty much everything that needed doing. Until the end of the 19th century, even senior consultants in prestigious teaching hospitals maintained general practices. Not only was it expected of them, but economics demanded it. By the First World War, scientific and clinical developments of the preceding generation

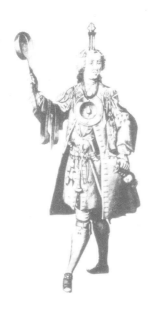

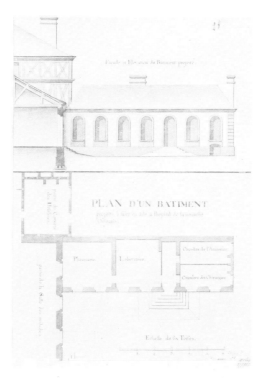

Far left: "A Surgeon or Barber." 18th century engraving by Martin Engelbrecht. [M.3.] *Left:* Plan for Building to Serve as Hospital of New Orleans. Ink and watercolor, 1737. [M.2.] Some believe this was the first real hospital in what is now the United States.

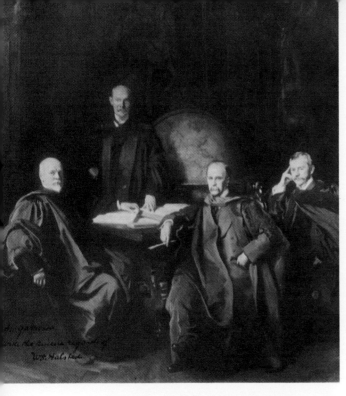

Above: The Founding Doctors of Johns Hopkins Medical School. Painting by John Singer Sargent, turn of the century. [N.L.M.] *Left to right:* William H. Welch, William Osler, W.S. Halsted and Howard Kelly. *Below:* Electro-Massage Machine. Engraving from *Harper's Weekly*, 1881. [N.Y.P.L./P.C.] The device, invented by Dr. John Butler of New York, was described as "especially salubrious in cases of rheumatism, nervous exhaustion, neuralgia and paralysis."

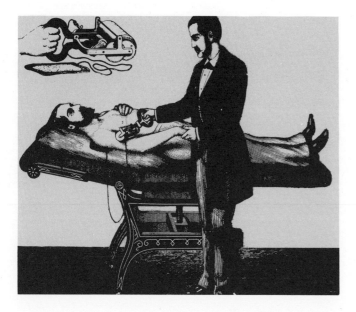

were complicated enough for the public to demand specialized knowledge and skills. Increasing numbers of physicians responded by limiting their practices to specialties. However, for most of the period covered by this book one man did everything—and people counted on him to do so.

Hospitals, as this book shows, were basically established to accommodate those whose own homes could not provide the most routine nursing care. Indeed, until about 1900, few people had anything done in a hospital. The physician's black bag carried drugs and instruments, and for the most part hospitals offered little more than what a doctor could provide in a patient's home. American medical practice was not hospital based or even office based until the First World War, simply because available technical resources were modest and easily transported. But technological changes began to proliferate; x-ray and laboratory diagnostic techniques grew exponentially, and soon demanded trained personnel and cumbersome, expensive equipment, most conveniently kept in hospitals. The result was that patients were transported to those hospitals. Thus not only did our "health care industry" begin, but the hospital acquired a new role. By 1920 one went to the hospital to get better, rather than in fear of dying.

Preoccupation with the divisiveness of the Civil War has too often led us to overlook its tremendous social and economic impact. Of enormous consequence, for instance, was the switch of mass production from military to civilian goods. Northern purveyors had discovered that soldiers could be successfully clothed from a limited, statistically determinable range of sizes in shoes, haberdashery and uniforms. The same principle of production held true for furniture, housewares, drugs, chemicals, and medical instruments. Once made by hand and to order, all these (and more) could be manufactured in quantity and sold from stock at competitive prices. Hence the American pharmaceutical industry burgeoned during the Civil War with the production of large quantities of standardized drugs of assayed potency. True, some of the goods were shoddy; nevertheless, mass production brought with it improved and more healthful living conditions for Americans.

Few of us are deluded by the notion that American women, or any other women for that matter, are passive creatures, inept in practical affairs and incapable of influencing economic and social policy. During the Civil War, women North and South kept things at home under control

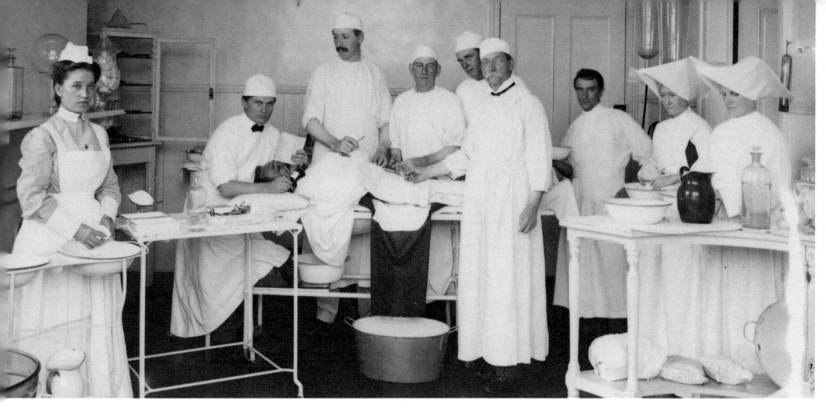

Operating Room, Mobile City Hospital, 1902. [H.M.P.S.] Drs. Howard, Frazer and Jackson demonstrating an operation for students.

and survived the loss of fathers, brothers, and sons. Out of the voluntary associations formed during the war for the relief of soldiers and their families emerged women's organizations dedicated to any number of specific community projects. For some time religious orders of women—Catholic, Lutheran, and Anglican—had founded hospitals and orphanages, but they received little credit, partially because most were Catholic and somehow not "American" enough, a judgment that would have surprised Sisters Elizabeth Bayly Seton, Catherine Drexel, and Cornelia Connolly! Between the Civil War and World War I, most of the institutions and organizations devoted to public health and welfare depended on the leadership of women, who were usually volunteers, but nonetheless effective, conscientious and persistent.

During most of the 1730 to 1930 period, the government did as little as possible, and through the better part of the 19th century, all that was needed to practice medicine was a diploma, or, in many places just the nerve to hang out a shingle. It was not until after 1900 that control of narcotics and dangerous drugs was seriously undertaken by the federal government; most medical specialty boards and colleges grew up between the First and Second World Wars.

Direct government provision of medical care was infrequent —a few Marine Hospitals, a few medical Officers of Health, and quarantine Officers constituted the government's largesse. Municipal almshouses and city hospitals existed chiefly in the Northeastern cities, and in many places, small tax levy appropriations were made to voluntary or Church-related hospitals to care for the indigent. But until the New Deal, government involvement in medical care was limited —very limited—and most people seemed to prefer *laissez-faire* to what would have been regarded as socialism.

This, then, is our introductory tour through two centuries. Much has changed, but more has not—mostly because people and their problems don't change very radically. Techniques, instruments, clothing, and interior decor may vary, but underneath, man is born, suffers, and dies. And the healing professions occasionally cure, often relieve, and always at least try to comfort.

William D. Sharpe, M.D.

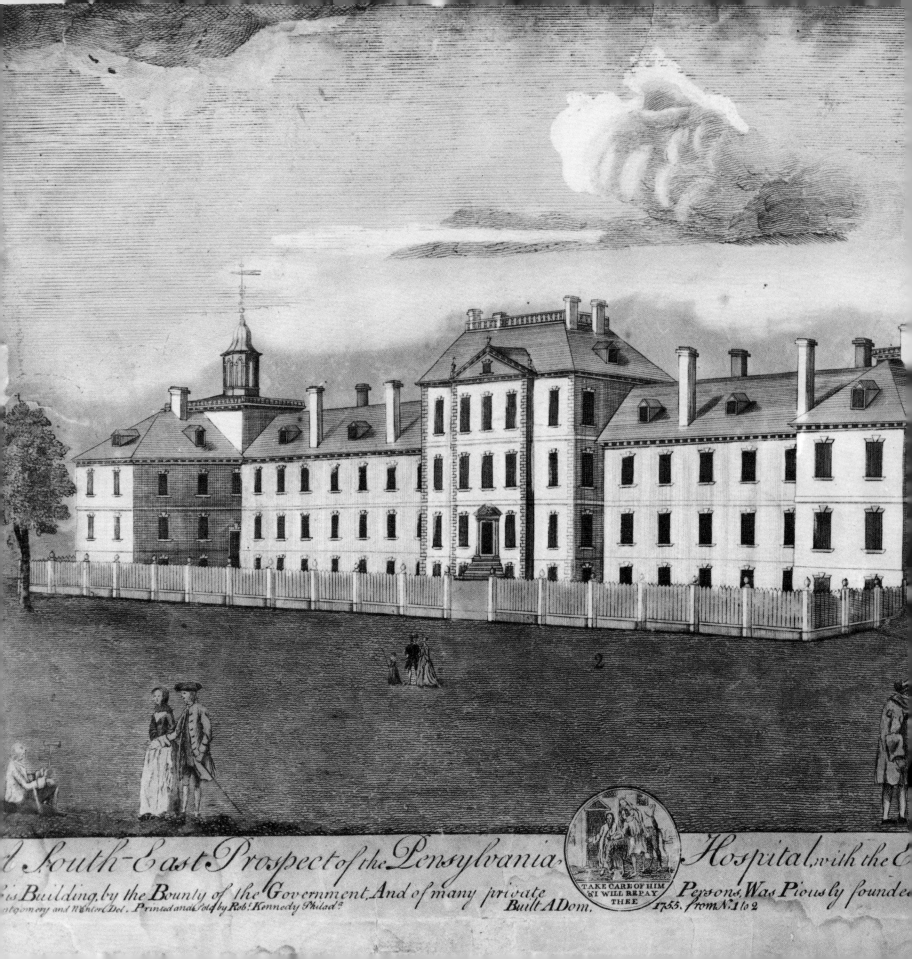

A South-East Prospect of the Pensylvania Hospital, with the E

is Building, by the Bounty of the Government, And of many private Persons, Was Piously founded

stgomery and Winter Del. Printed and Sold by Robt. Kennedy Philada.   Built A Dom. 1755. from No. 1 to 2

TAKE CARE OF HIM & I WILL REPAY THEE

CHAPTER ONE

1730-1779

Benjamin Franklin's cherished goal, the founding of Pennsylvania Hospital, was officially realized in May, 1751 when a bill was enacted in Pennsylvania stating: ". . . the Relief of the Sick Poor is not only an Act of Humanity, but a religious Duty; . . . there are frequently, in many parts of this Province, poor distemp'rd Persons, who languish long in Pain and Misery under various Disorders of Body and Mind . . . which Inconveniency might be happily removed, by collecting the Patients into one common Provincial Hospital . . . where they may be comfortably subsisted, and their Health taken Care of at a small Charge."

The founding of Pennsylvania Hospital launched a new era in American medicine. Indeed, the disorderly and inadequate colonial "hospitals," essentially workhouses and houses of correction (where wardens were often permitted to fetter or shackle, moderately whip, and even starve their inmates), gradually became institutions of time past.

Pennsylvania Hospital represented a significant step toward the practice of medicine in a free and egalitarian society—in short, American society. As Franklin wrote in the August, 1751 *Pennsylvania Gazette*: In America ". . . a Beggar, in a well regulated Hospital stands an equal Chance with a [European] Prince in his Palace for a comfortable subsistence, and expeditious and effectual Cure of His Diseases."

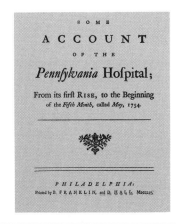

Left: Pennsylvania Hospital. Engraving, c. 1780. [P.H.] America's first general hospital. *Above:* An account of its founding printed by Benjamin Franklin. 1754. [P.H.]

1732: Hat Act restricted colonial industry

1732-57: Benjamin Franklin's *Poor Richard's Almanack* published

1733: Georgia, last of 13 colonies, founded
Molasses Act restricted colonial trade

1734: Protestants emigrated to Georgia from Austria

1741: Alaskan mainland discovered by Vitus Bering

1744-48: King George's War

1744-54: Virginians and Pennsylvanians moved West

1752: Franklin invented lightning rod

1730   1740   1750

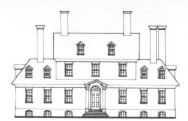

Friends Almshouse, Philadelphia

1732: The Friends' Almshouse was erected in Philadelphia. This was a poorhouse, not a hospital, but its infirmary cared for paupers who were ill or insane. Dr. William Shippen, Sr. (1712-1801), apothecary and physician, is believed to have been the first doctor associated with it. By the late 1700s, the infirmary grew, and began its evolution into the Philadelphia General Hospital.

1734: A "Publick Workhouse and House of Correction," including an infirmary which later developed into Bellevue Hospital, was commissioned by New York City. This almshouse was built in 1736, and in 1811 the establishment—containing a ward for the sick as well as a penitentiary and church school—acquired its present site at Bell Vue Place. It was enlarged by a new "fever hospital" after the yellow fever epidemic of 1819, and assumed the name Bellevue Hospital in 1825.

1735—The hitherto mild disease of diphtheria assumed a fatal form in an outbreak in Kingston, New Hampshire, where all of its first forty victims died.

1736: St. Philip's Hospital in Charleston, South Carolina, was founded. Built for the paupers of St. Philip's parish, this institution was primarily a workhouse and penitentiary as well as a hospital for the indigent sick. It was no longer in existence by the end of the century.

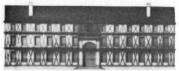

Royal Hospital, New Orleans

1737: The Royal (later Charity) Hospital in New Orleans was established. Founded by the French in territory that did not become part of the United States until the Louisiana Purchase, this institution became, in 1803, the third public general hospital in this country.

1741: Yellow fever struck Philadelphia. The ill were housed in a pesthouse on League Island. In epidemics like this, mortality rates often reached 85 percent. Preventive medicine, introduced with the 1721 smallpox inoculations by Zabdiel Boylston (1679-1766) of Boston, was inadequate to control yellow fever until the 20th century.

1742: A post mortem examination done by Thomas Cadwalader of Philadelphia is credited as being the first scientific autopsy performed in the territory that later became the United States.

1745: The unusual specialty of a physician who was one of the first obstetricians received comment in his obituary. When John Dupuy, M.D., of New York, died in the prime of life, the newspaper noted that he was "a man midwife," and added, "There is none like him."

1750: The first recorded instruction in anatomy by dissection took place in the infirmary in the New York City almshouse (later Bellevue Hospital). An executed criminal was dissected for students by Dr. John Bard (1716-1799).

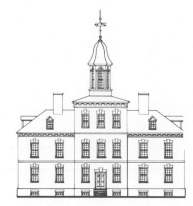

Pennsylvania Hospital, Philadelphia, 1751

1751: Pennsylvania Hospital, the first general hospital in the United States, was founded in Philadelphia. Established through the efforts of Benjamin Franklin and Dr. Thomas Bond, the hospital opened in 1752 —the oldest institution intended solely for the care of the sick and wounded in territory that is now the United States (some hospitals in Canada and Mexico can claim to be older). From its beginning, the hospital also cared for the insane.

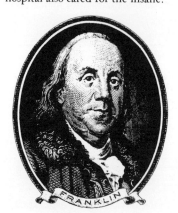

Benjamin Franklin

1752: First hospital pharmacy opened in the Pennsylvania Hospital. The first pharmacist was Jonathan Roberts. His successor, the pharmacist-physician Dr. John Morgan, played an important role in the development of professional pharmacy in North America.

14

1754-63: French and Indian Wars

1760: Estimated population of 13 colonies, 1,600,000

1764: French founded St. Louis
Sugar Act passed

1765: Stamp Act passed; colonies protested

1766: Stamp Act repealed by Parliament

1767: Townshend Acts restricted importation into colonies

1768: Colonies protested Townshend Acts
British troops in Boston

1770: Boston Massacre; Five Bostonians killed

1773: Boston Tea Party

1774: Parliament passed Intolerable Acts
First Continental Congress held

1775: Battles of Lexington, Concord, Bunker Hill
Washington named commander-in-chief

1776: Declaration of Independence

1777: *The Stars and Stripes* adopted by Congress
Winter: Ordeal of Valley Forge

1779: John Paul Jones on the *Bonhomme Richard* defeated *Serapis*

1760   1770   1779

1753: Benjamin Franklin's *Experiments in Electricity* was published. Sponsored by the English Quaker, Dr. John Fothergill (1712-1780), this work spurred interest in possible applications of electricity to medicine. Franklin experimented on victims of palsy, but honestly admitted he observed no physical changes in paralyzed patients.

1760: The first law requiring medical practitioners to obtain licenses from a board of examiners was passed in New York. In 1772 New Jersey enacted a similar law.

1762: Pioneering lectures in anatomy and midwifery were given in Philadelphia by Dr. William Shippen, Jr. (1736-1808). Shippen, recently graduated from Edinburgh, used life-sized anatomical drawings donated by Dr. John Fothergill and plaster models to demonstrate childbirth. When he showed specimens from human dissections, angry mobs threatened him for grave-robbing.

1763: Smallpox was used as a biological weapon in the last year of the French and Indian Wars. Lord Jeffrey Amherst (1717-1797), British captor of Louisburg, Ticonderoga and Montreal, ordered blankets infected with smallpox to be distributed among Indian tribes supporting the French. Smallpox was prevalent throughout the colonies, particularly in the following decade.

1765: The first medical school in the United States was organized in Philadelphia. Dr. John Morgan (1735-1789), persuaded the College of Philadelphia (later the University of Pennsylvania) to set up a medical faculty.

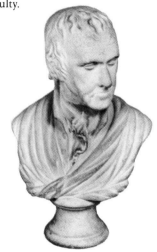

Dr. Benjamin Rush

Morgan taught theory and practice of medicine, while Dr. William Shippen, Jr. taught anatomy and surgery. In 1769 Dr. Benjamin Rush (1745-1813) joined them as professor of chemistry. Shippen later claimed that Morgan had stolen his ideas for the school, and bitter rivalry developed between them. Rush and Shippen quarreled during the Revolutionary War, when Rush was surgeon general and Shippen was director general of the army's medical services.

1766: The New Jersey Medical Society was formed, one of several state associations dating from colonial years. American medical practitioners revived the system of the British guilds, regulating their fees and practices. Members of the New Jersey society agreed to charge a minimum of 25 cents for a country call, depending upon mileage traveled, and as much as $3.50 for delivering a baby.

1768: King's College in New York City established a medical department. The moving spirit behind this new school, and its first professor of physic, was young Dr. Samuel Bard, who also helped found New York Hospital in 1771.

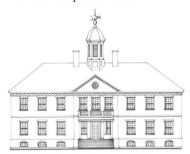

Eastern Asylum for the Insane, Williamsburg

1768: Insane Hospital at Williamsburg, Virginia, was established. Apart from the Pennsylvania Hospital, this was the only American institution significantly devoted to the care of mental patients in this century.

1775: Joseph Warren (1741-1775), Boston physician and political leader, was killed in the battle of Bunker Hill. Warren was the patriot who dispatched Paul Revere and William Dawes to warn Concord that the British were coming. Warren's descendants were leaders in New England medicine for generations.

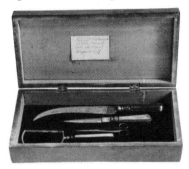

Military Surgeon's Kit, 1777

1776: Inoculation of all soldiers in the Continental Army was ordered by George Washington. At this time an estimated 3,500 physicians were practicing medicine in the colonies that became the United States: fewer than 400 of them held university degrees; the rest had learned through apprenticeship.

1778: First American pharmacopoeia was published in Philadelphia. This small booklet, a landmark in the history of American pharmacy, was called the *Lititz Pharmacopoeia* after Lititz, Pennsylvania, where an army hospital housed wounded patriots.

15

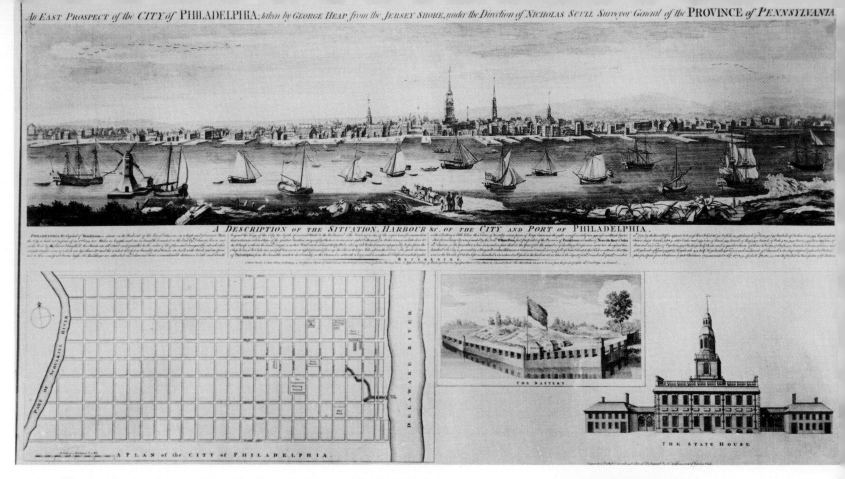

A DESCRIPTION of the SITUATION, HARBOUR &c. of the CITY and PORT of PHILADELPHIA.

A PLAN of the CITY of PHILADELPHIA.

THE BATTERY

THE STATE HOUSE

Philadelphia, from the New Jersey Shore. Engraving, 1754. [L.P.C.] William Penn's Quaker "City of Brotherly Love," was the fastest-growing city in the British Empire in size, population and wealth.

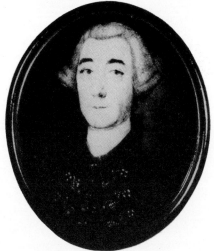

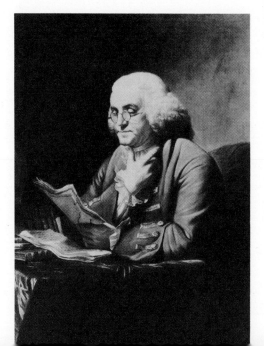

Left: Benjamin Franklin. Painting, 18th century. [P.C.] Inventor, statesman, and co-founder of Pennsylvania Hospital. *Above:* Dr. Thomas Bond. Miniature painting, 18th century. [P.C.P.S.] Co-founder of Pennsylvania Hospital.

16

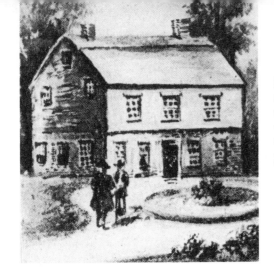

Pennsylvania Hospital, 1752. Print, 19th century. [P.H.] After its founding in 1751, the hospital was temporarily housed in a private residence. It was the first hospital on these shores to care for both charity cases and paying private patients.

Above: Admission Slip Signed by Benjamin Franklin, June 4, 1753. Pen and ink. [P.H.] Franklin wrote to "Sister" Elizabeth, who was responsible for Pennsylvania Hospital's admissions. *Right:* Abstract of Cases Admitted from February, 1752 through April, 1754. Print, 1754. [P.H.] Listed are some of the maladies then prevalent. Ague: malarial fever; Dropsies: edema, an abnormal accumulation of fluid; Scorbutick: related to scurvy, spongy gums, loosening of teeth due to Vitamin C deficiency; Ulcers, with Caries: probably included external sores, possibly those caused by social diseases, and osteomyelitis, especially of teeth.

[36]

ABSTRACT of Cases admitted into the Pennsylvania Hospital, from the Eleventh of the Second Month, 1752, to the Twenty-seventh of the Fourth Month, 1754.

	Admitted.	Cured.	Relieved.	Irregular Behaviour.	Incurable.	Taken away by their Friends.	Dead.	Remaining.
AGUES	3	3	—	—	—	—	—	—
Cancer,	3	2	—	—	—	—	—	1
Colliquative Purging,	2	—	—	—	—	—	2	—
Consumption,	1	—	—	—	—	1	—	—
Contusion,	1	1	—	—	—	—	—	1
Cough, of long standing,	1	1	—	—	—	—	—	—
Dropsies,	9	4	1	—	—	—	3	—
Empyema,	1	1	—	—	—	—	—	—
Eyes disordered,	2	1	1	—	—	—	—	—
Falling Sickness,	3	1	—	—	2	—	—	—
Fevers,	2	2	—	—	—	—	—	—
Fistula in *Ano*,	3	2	1	—	—	—	—	—
—— in *Perinæo*,	2	1	—	—	—	—	—	1
Flux,	1	1	—	—	—	—	1	—
Gutta Serena,	1	1	—	—	—	—	—	—
Hair Lip,	1	—	—	—	—	—	—	1
Hypocondriac Melancholy,	1	—	—	—	—	—	—	1
Hypopyon,	1	1	—	—	—	—	—	—
Lunacy,	18	2	3	—	4	6	—	3
Mortification,	1	—	—	—	—	—	1	—
Prolapsus *Ani*,	1	1	—	—	—	—	—	—
—— *Uteri*,	1	1	—	—	—	—	—	—
Palsy,	1	1	—	—	—	—	—	—
—— of the Bladder,	1	—	—	—	—	—	—	1
Rheumatism and Sciatica,	6	4	—	—	—	—	—	2
Scorbutick and scrophulous Diseases,	9	6	1	1	—	—	—	1
Ulcers, with Caries, &c. ——	37	21	4	2	1	—	3	3
Vertigo,	1	1	4	—	—	3	3	3
Uterine Disorder,	1	1	—	—	—	—	—	—
Wen,	1	1	—	—	—	—	—	—
Wounded,	1	1	—	—	—	—	—	—
In all,	117	60	11	3	7	10	10	16

N. B. THE Majority of the Lunaticks taken in had been many Years disorder'd, and their Diseases become too habitual to admit of Relief; others whose Cases were recent, and might probably have been cured, being put in at private Expence, were so hastily taken away by their Friends, that sufficient Time was not allowed for their Recovery: The Managers have therefore, as well for the Sake of the Afflicted, as the Reputation of the Hospital, resolved to admit none hereafter, who are not allowed to remain twelve Months in the House, if not cured sooner, or judged by the Physicians to be incurable.

THE Choice of the Sick to be supported on the publick Stock, was confined to such only whose Cases could not be healed properly in their respective Habitations, but required the extraordinary Conveniences and Advantages of an Hospital; amongst these, several, for want of this noble Charity in Time, had languished too long to receive any other Advantage from it than the Relief of their Poverty, and the Satisfaction of being convinced they had every Chance for Recovery that Care and Tenderness could afford.

FROM

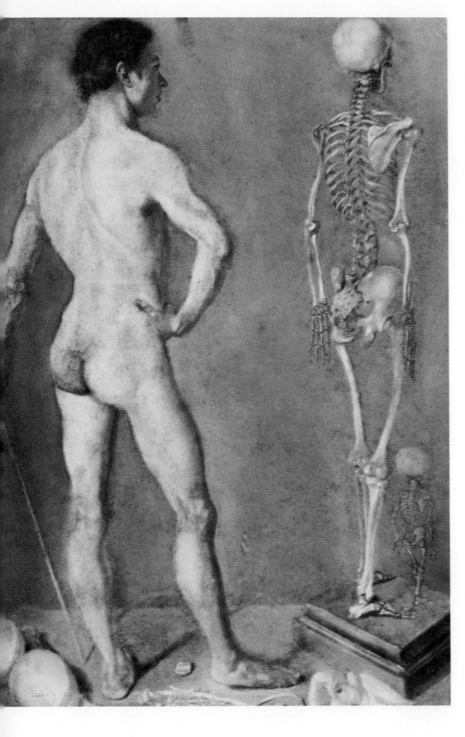

Left and far right on facing page: Anatomical Paintings. 18th century. [P.H.] Presented to Pennsylvania Hospital in 1762 by Dr. John Fothergill of London to further the teaching of medicine in the colonies. *Below:* Dr. John Fothergill. Wedgewood Jasperware minature, 18th century. [P.C.P.S.] Dr. Fothergill, a leading Quaker philanthropist of London, instructed a number of Americans who studied medicine in England.

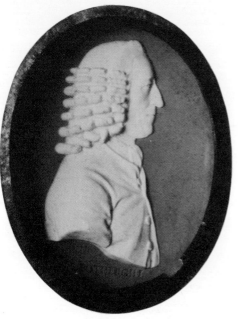

Amputation of a Leg. Watercolor, English, 18th century. [M.5.] A demonstration in a surgical amphitheater before medical students. Though the illustration may be somewhat exaggerated, the absence of anesthesia and aseptic conditions is clear. Note the presence of the black student, perhaps from a West Indian colony.

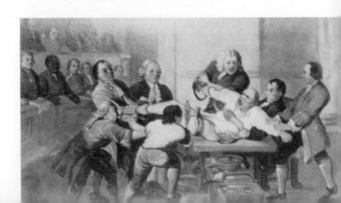

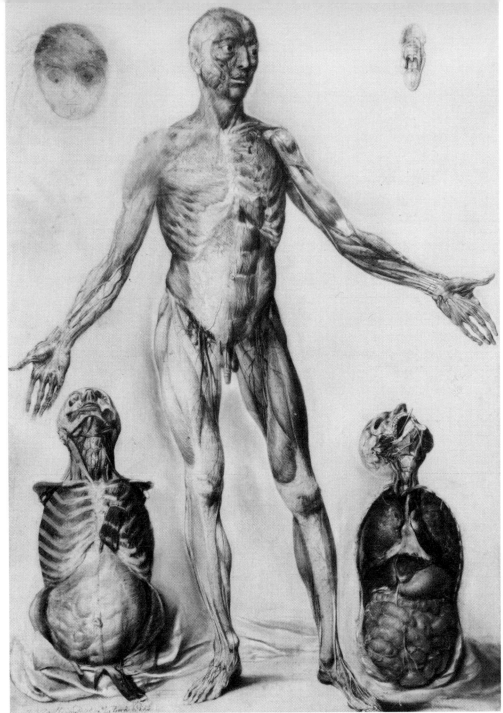

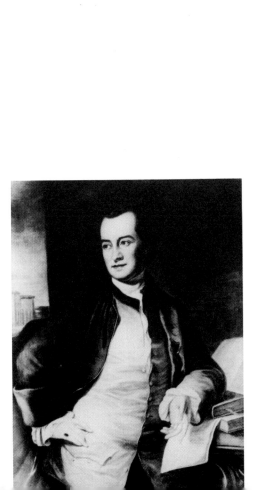

Left: John Morgan, M.D. Painting, 18th century. [P.H.] Morgan was a
member of the first graduating class of what is now the University of
Pennsylvania, and a 1763 graduate of Edinburgh University's medical
school. Returning to Philadelphia, he served as the second Apothecary
at Pennsylvania Hospital and in 1765 was a founder of the School of
Medicine of the University of Pennsylvania.

19

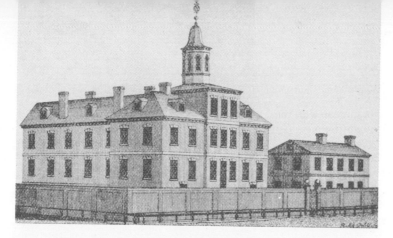

Above: Pennsylvania Hospital with 1768 Elaboratory Addition. Print, 19th century. [P.H.] From its earliest days, the hospital employed an apprentice whose role was "to learn the Art, Trade and Mystery of an Apothecare." *Right:* Title Page: Lititz Pharmacopoeia. Print, 1778. [L.C.P.] This first authoritative American listing of drugs, chemicals and medicinal preparations was formulated in 1778.

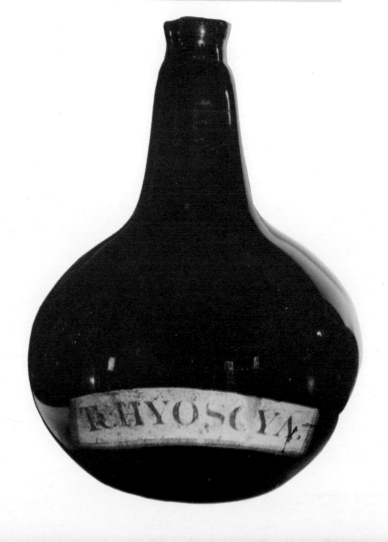

PHARMACOPOEIA

SIMPLICIORUM

ET

EFFICACIORUM,

IN USUM

NOSOCOMII MILITARIS,

AD EXERCITUM

Fœderatarum *Americæ* Civitatum

PERTINENTIS;

HODIERNÆ NOSTRÆ INOPIÆ RERUMQUE
ANGUSTIIS,

Feroci hostium sævitiæ, belloque crudeli ex inopinatò
patriæ nostræ illato debitis,

MAXIME ACCOMMODATA.

PHILADELPHIÆ:

Ex Officina STYNER & CIST. M DCC LXXVIII.

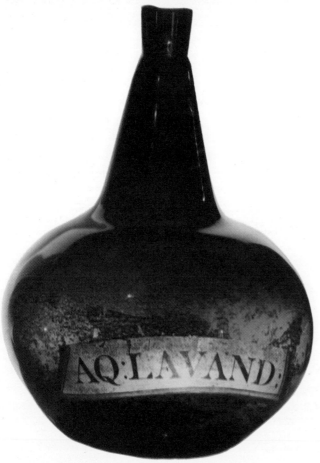

Apothecary Bottles. Glass, 18th century. [A.P.A.] *Left:* Lavand was lavender water, used to relieve indigestion and as a perfume. *Right:* Tincture of Hyoscyamus (henbane), was used as a sedative and to cure spasms.

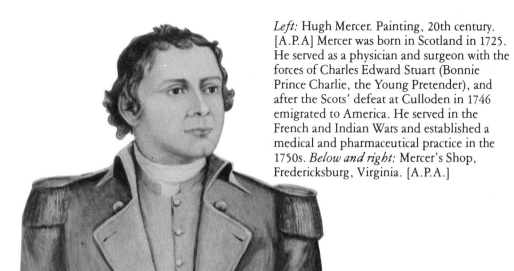

Left: Hugh Mercer. Painting, 20th century. [A.P.A] Mercer was born in Scotland in 1725. He served as a physician and surgeon with the forces of Charles Edward Stuart (Bonnie Prince Charlie, the Young Pretender), and after the Scots' defeat at Culloden in 1746 emigrated to America. He served in the French and Indian Wars and established a medical and pharmaceutical practice in the 1750s. *Below and right:* Mercer's Shop, Fredericksburg, Virginia. [A.P.A.]

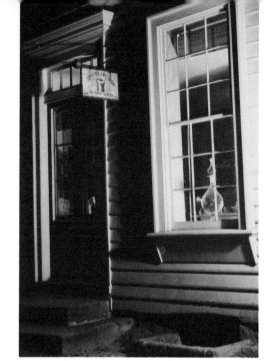

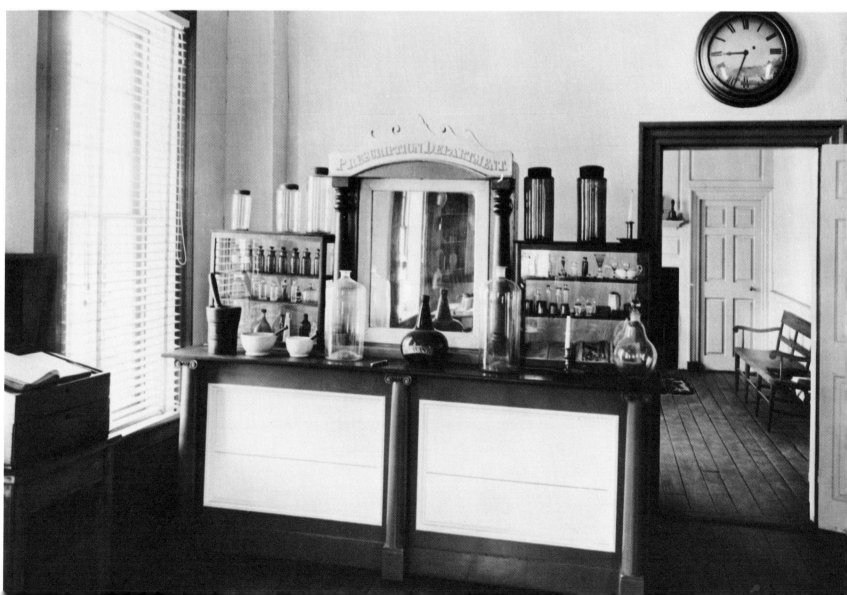

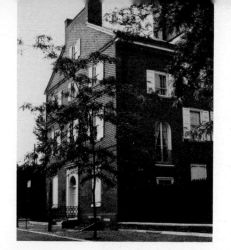

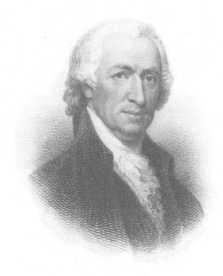

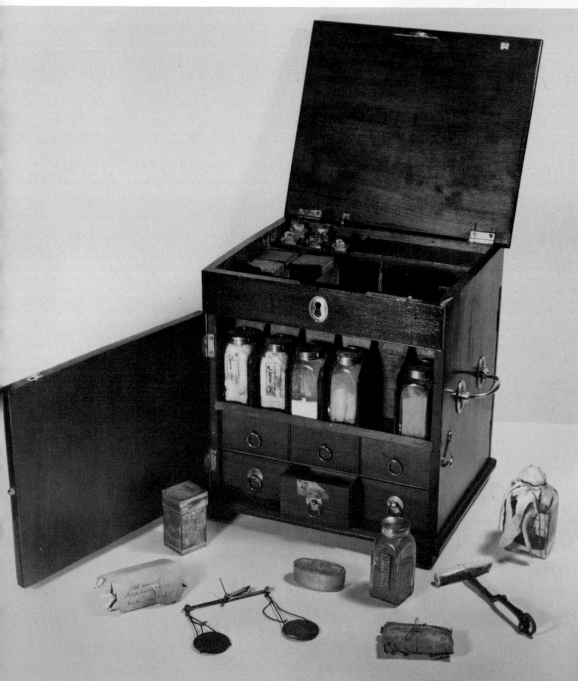

Above: William Shippen Jr. Engraving, 18th century. [N.L.M.] Like his father, William Shippen, who began his professional life as a pharmacist in the 1730s, Shippen Jr. was elected to "the faculty," or attending staff, at Pennsylvania Hospital. *Above left:* The Shippen House. Photograph, 20th century. [S.K.C.] *Left:* Medicine Chest. Mahogany, 18th century. [P.C.P.S.] William Shippen Jr.'s chest contained medicine, an apothecary scale, and, *right foreground,* a toothkey for extracting teeth.

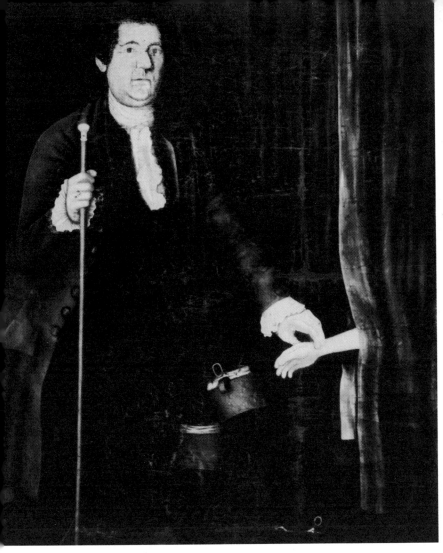

Dr. William Clysson. Painting, 18th century. [M.6.] Dr. Clysson is shown taking the pulse of his obviously modest female patient. Colonial physicians like this New Englander adopted the style of London practitioners who carried a gold-headed cane as a symbol of their profession.

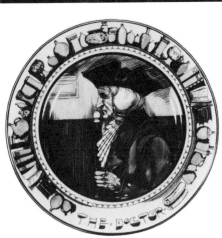

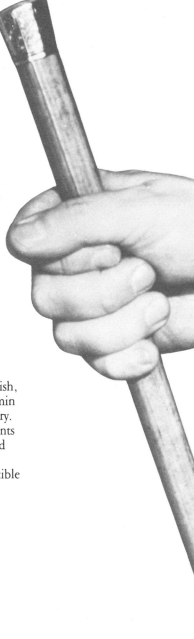

Left: The Physician. Porcelain plate, English, 19th century. [P.C.P.S.] *Right:* Dr. Benjamin Rush's Cane. Wood and gold, 18th century. [P.C.P.S.] Dr. Rush admonished his students at the Medical School that affectations and pompousness—as seen in the Londoner portrayed on the plate— were "incompatible with the simplicity of science."

23

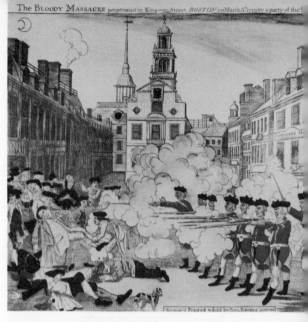

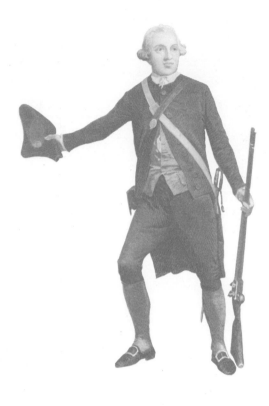

Above: General Joseph Warren. Engraving, 18th century. [L.C.] The renowned Boston physician. *Above right:* The Boston Massacre. Engraving, 1770. [P.C.] Paul Revere engraved this famous broadside. *Right:* Death of General Joseph Warren. Painting by John Trumbull, 18th century. [L.C.]

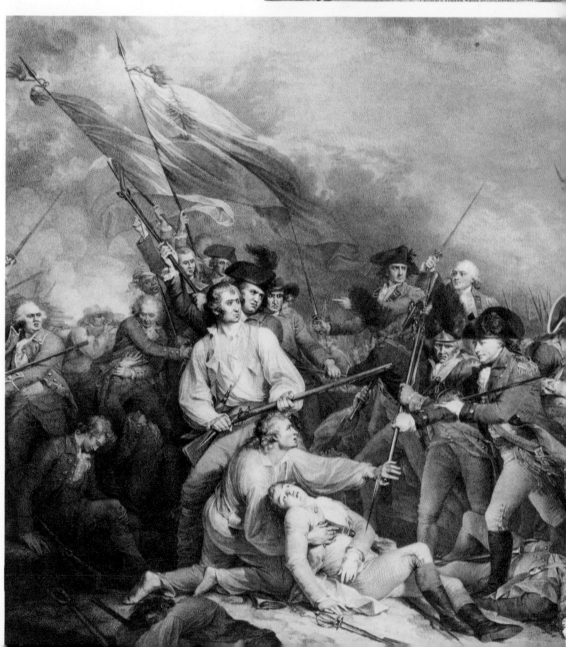

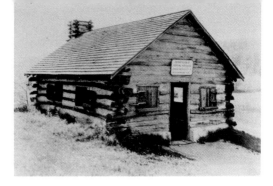

Above: Reproduction of Hospital Hut. Photograph, 20th century. [N.L.M.] This reproduction at Valley Forge, Pa., is on the original site of the hospital for Washington's army in the cruel winter of 1777–78. *Right:* Medicine Chest. Wood and brass, 18th century. [V.F.H.S.] Some patriotic Philadelphia physicians served at Valley Forge, where this chest is known to have been used.

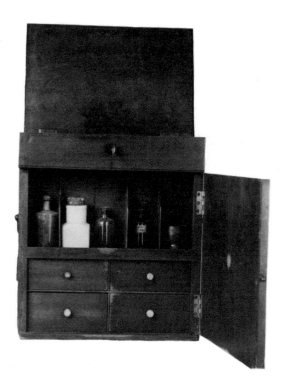

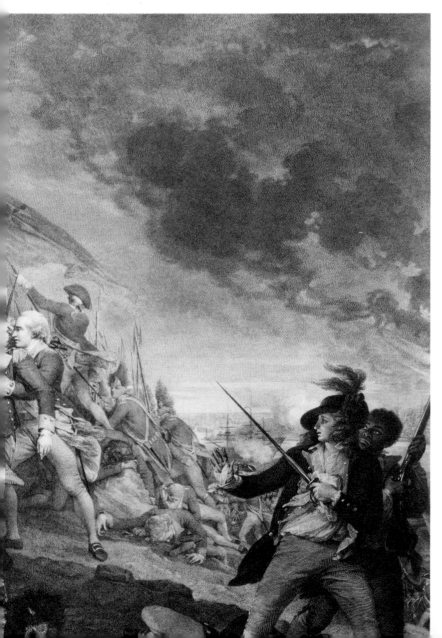

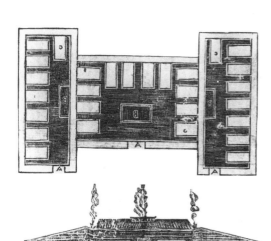

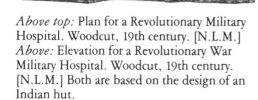

Above top: Plan for a Revolutionary Military Hospital. Woodcut, 19th century. [N.L.M.] *Above:* Elevation for a Revolutionary War Military Hospital. Woodcut, 19th century. [N.L.M.] Both are based on the design of an Indian hut.

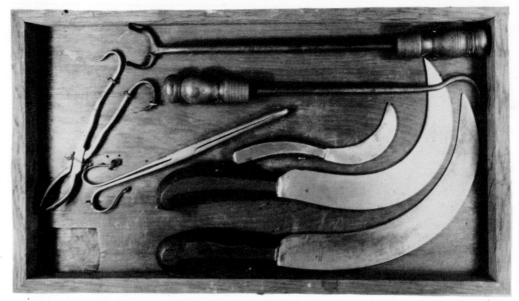

Left: Surgical Kit Used During The Revolutionary War. [D.O.A.] *Below:* Medical Kit. Miscellaneous materials, 18th century. [D.O.A.] This medical kit was used by Dr. Solomon Drowne of the Continental Army. Its contents include drugs, scissors, scalpels, curved needles, suture material, a pharmaceutical scale and weights, and a leg splint.

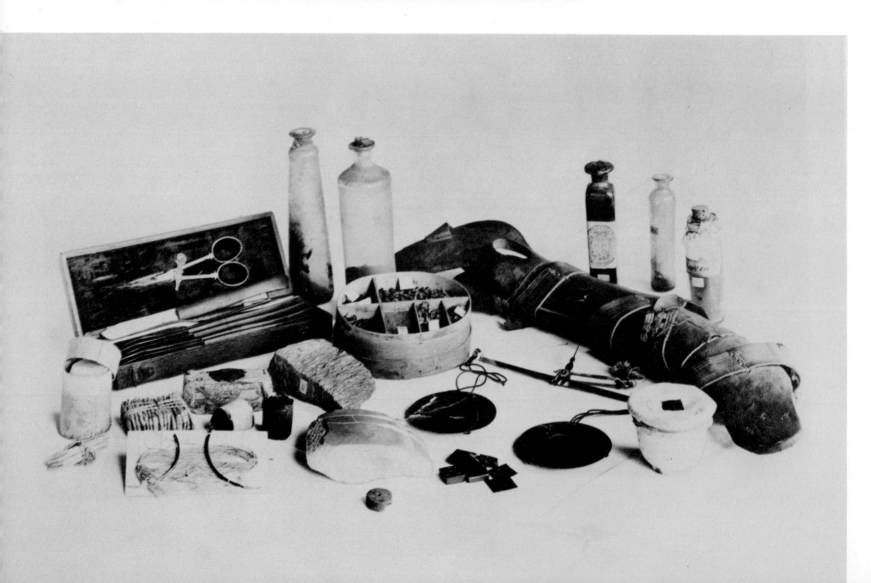

Advertisement for Mary Bass, Midwife, from the *Essex* (Mass.) *Gazette.* July 14-21, 1772. Print, [N.Y.P.L./P.C.] In 1789, another midwife, Grace Mulligan, began practice in Delaware after studying with "Dr. Shippen Jr. of Philadelphia [for] better than a year."

Above: Military Surgeon's Kit. Miscellaneous materials, 18th century. [H.M.S.] The contents of the kit of Dr. Peter Turner, surgeon of the 1st Rhode Island Regiment, were curved and straight amputating knives and a small saw. *Right:* Easy Chair . . . "useful for lying-in women and sick persons." Engraving, 1793. [L.C.P.] In this period, the medical care of pregnant women was largely in the hands of midwives, who ideally possessed "slender hands, long fingers, tender feelings, sympathy," and would be "helpful and above all, silent."

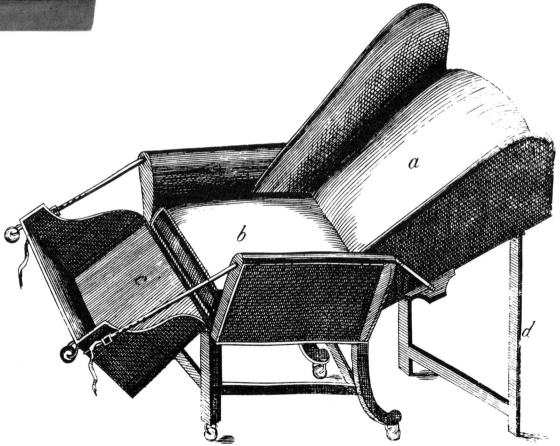

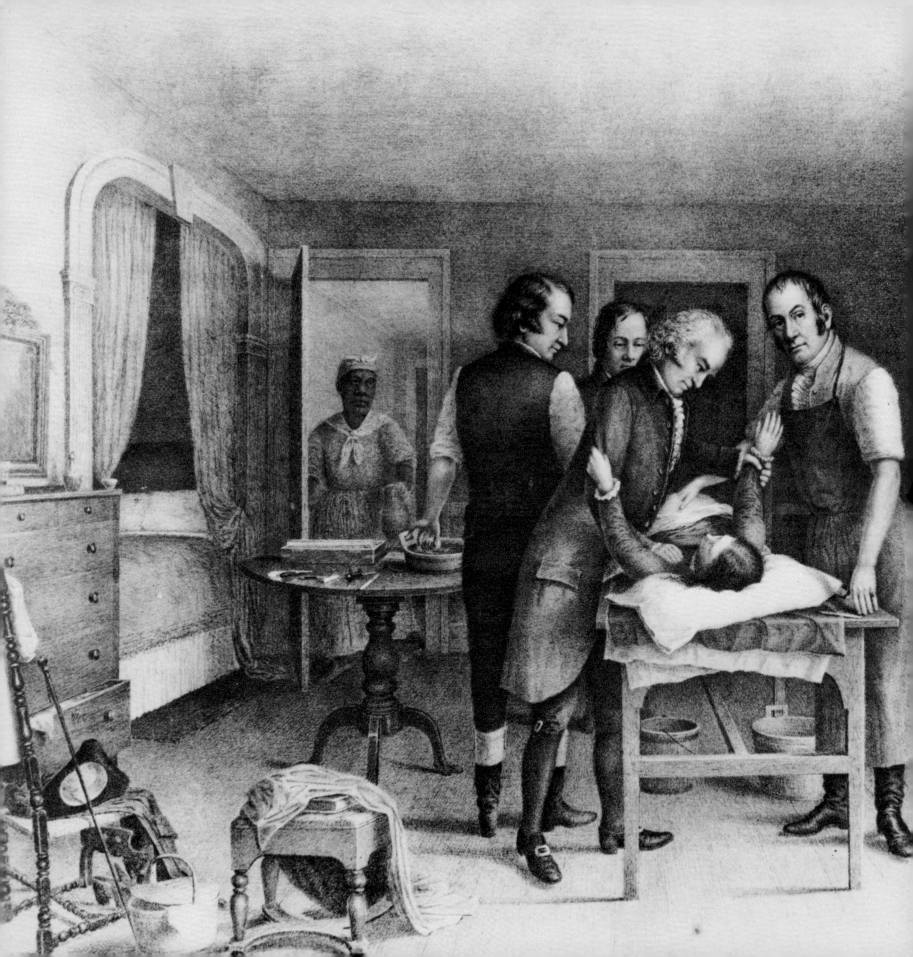

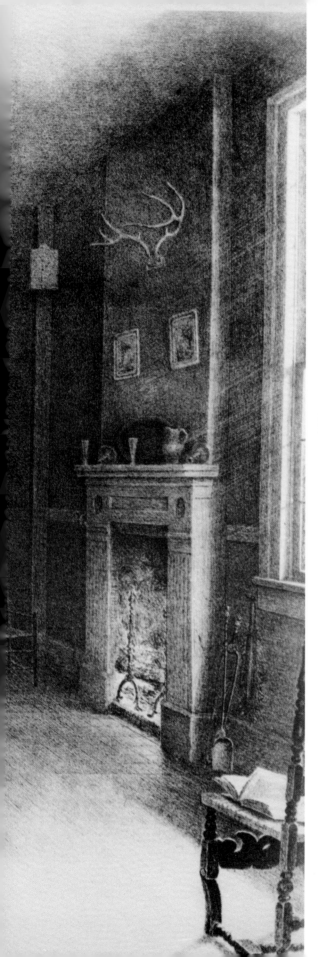

CHAPTER TWO

1780-1819

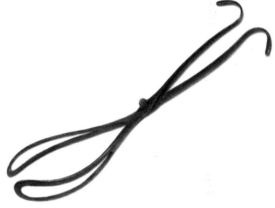

O n November 8, 1783, in a letter to Dr. John Warren, Professor of Anatomy and Surgery, Harvard University's President, Joseph Willard, voiced grave misgivings about Harvard Medical School's initial success: "I have been expecting some time past to see an advertisement from the Medical Professors in the Newspapers. I should think that if they begin their lectures this fall, as I hope they will, that the sooner they advertise the better. They will not be able to know till they advertise what number of the students in physic will be likely to attend them . . .

"I hope it will not be long before the profession advertise, lest the public begin to think that the proceedings of the University were mere parade, and that the medical institution was likely to be attended with no utility. The students in physic will not, I suppose, be numerous this season; but I doubt not, if these lectures should meet with approbation . . . the profession will in a year or two find their pupils so increased that their labors will not be without emolument."

The aim of Harvard Medical School and those that followed in the new republic was to upgrade general medical standards and rid the profession of the "inhuman barbarians," the ill-trained and untrained physicians of the colonial period. As criteria for admission and graduation became more stringent, American medical institutions presented a serious challenge to their European counterparts.

Left: First Ovariotomy, by Dr. Ephraim McDowell. Lithograph, 19th century. [L.C.] The operation was the most celebrated surgical feat by a frontier doctor in the annals of American medicine. *Above:* Forceps, Metal. European, 18th century. [N.L.M.]

1780: Benedict Arnold declared a traitor
Inflation blanketed country
1781: Bank of North America incorporated
Articles of Confederation ratified
1782: British surrendered at Yorktown
British agreed to recognize U.S. independence
1783: U.S. and Britain signed peace treaty
Webster published *The American Spelling Book*
1784-87: Economy in depression

1785: Law established national coinage

1787: Constitutional Convention convened;
George Washington presided
1787-88: States ratified Constitution
1787-88: Hamilton, Madison, Jay wrote
The Federalist Papers

1789: Washington inaugurated President
Supreme Court created
1790: First U.S. census; 3,929,214 inhabitants
1791: Vermont became 14th state
Bill of Rights adopted
1792: Kentucky became 15th state
Washington and John Adams reelected
1793: Eli Whitney invented cotton gin
1794: Whiskey Rebellion
1795: Naturalization Act
1796: Washington's Farewell Address
John Adams elected President
Tennessee became 16th state
1798: The Department of Navy
created
1799: George
Washington died

1780

1790

1781: Medical Society of Massachusetts was founded. In 1790 it began to publish proceedings.

1782: Harvard University medical department founded. The school opened officially in 1783. John Warren, Benjamin Waterhouse and Aaron Dexter formed the three-man faculty, teaching without benefit of any hospital affiliation. Warren taught anatomy and surgery, Waterhouse theory and practice of physic, and Dexter, chemistry and materia medica.

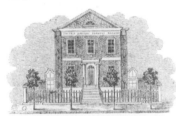

The Philadelphia Dispensary

1786: The Philadelphia Dispensary was instituted, the first free dispensary in the United States. The organizing physician was Dr. Benjamin Rush (1745?-1813), signer of the Declaration of Independence, a popular professor of medicine and chemistry, founder of the first American antislavery society, and the leading physician of his time. Rush, who practiced from 1769 to 1813, was the first American doctor to win world fame. He trained as many as 3,000 American physicians, and his lasting contributions include therapy for the mentally ill.

1787: The College of Physicians of Philadelphia was founded. Dr. John Redman (1722-1808), esteemed older colleague of Morgan, Shippen and Rush, was elected president annually until 1804, when he was allowed to retire at his own request. The College began publishing proceedings in 1793.

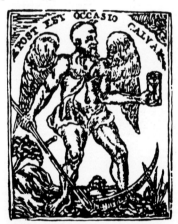

The Angel of Death, Detail of Mortality Report

1788: In the Doctors' Riot, angry New Yorkers attacked New York Hospital and seized four physicians suspected of grave robbing. Guilty of nothing worse than dissecting a corpse, the four anatomists were rescued and released. All the Hospital's doctors had to hide or leave town until the rumors subsided.

1789: The first widespread epidemic of influenza attacked the U.S.

1790: Benjamin Rush estimated that of one hundred people born then in Philadelphia, at the end of:

Years	Survived	Years	Survived
6	64	46	10
16	46	56	6
26	26	66	3
36	16	76	1

1791: New York Hospital, established 20 years earlier, began to function in full. The first buildings of the hospital, chartered in 1771, were destroyed by fire as they were nearing completion in 1775. The hospital accommodated up to 60 patients, segregated by sex and race, and had a mortality rate of one in twenty. Patients paid $2 per week.

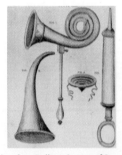

Plate from Bell's A System of Surgery

1791: The first American edition of Benjamin Bell's *A System of Surgery* was published. Bell was the first surgeon at the Edinburgh Infirmary, Scotland, a city in which many American physicians received their training. The American edition of his work was published in Worcester, Massachusetts.

1793: Yellow fever struck Philadelphia. This was the start of a 12-year epidemic that spread from the Northeast to the South. Ten percent of Philadelphia's population died. One hero of the plague was Benjamin Rush. On the theory that most illnesses were forms of fever caused by over-stimulated blood vessels, Rush believed that withdrawing 50 ounces of blood could save a patient's life.

1796: Boston Dispensary was established.

1798: The medical department of Dartmouth College was founded. For the first ten years, Nathan Smith was its one-man faculty. With its opening, four medical schools— the others were in Philadelphia, New York and Boston—taught the nation's physicians.

1798: The Marine Hospital Service was created by Act of Congress. The first federal government office concerned with health began operating hospitals for disabled seamen. In the same year, George Balfour was appointed the first United States Navy surgeon.

1798: Pioneer compilation of American plant drugs was issued by Benjamin Smith Barton.

1799: The first lying-in wards in the United States were opened at Bellevue Hospital, New York City.

00: 5,308,000 inhabitants; 3.8% urban, 96.2% rural

Capitol transferred to Washington

1801: Thomas Jefferson elected President

1802: U.S. Military Academy opened

1803: Louisiana Purchase

Ohio became 17th state

1804: Hamilton killed by Burr in duel

Jefferson reelected

1804-06: Lewis and Clark expedition

1807: Aaron Burr tried

Embargo Act

First trip of Robert Fulton's steamboat

1808: Importation of slaves outlawed

James Madison elected President

1810: 7,239,000 inhabitants reported

1811: Indians defeated in Battle of Tippecanoe

1812: Madison reelected President

War of 1812

Louisiana became 18th state

1813: War with Creek Indians

1814: British burned Washington

Treaty of Ghent ended War of 1812

Francis Scott Key wrote *The Star-Spangled Banner*

1815: Battle of Waterloo

1816: Indiana became 19th state

James Monroe elected President

1817: Mississippi became 20th state

Construction of Erie Canal began

1818: Illinois became 21st state

1819: Alabama became 22nd state

Nation's first major banking crisis

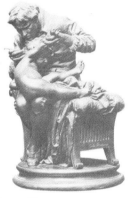

Sculpture of Dr. Jenner Inoculating His Son

1800: Dr. Benjamin Waterhouse (1754-1846), introduced vaccination as a general practice to America, leading to the control of smallpox. More than 50 epidemics had scourged colonial North America. The English physician Edward Jenner (1749-1823), demonstrated in 1796 that scraping or rubbing cowpox virus into the skin would produce antibodies against smallpox. Inoculation had been used by Zabdiel Boylston and others, but Waterhouse was the first American physician to establish it generally.

1803: Dr. Edward Jenner received an honorary degree from Harvard University.

1803: The Charity Hospital of New Orleans, established 1737, became the third general public hospital in the United States after the Louisiana Purchase.

1805: Dr. Philip Syng Physick was appointed to the Chair of Surgery at the University of Pennsylvania Medical School. Trained by John Hunter of Scotland and granted an M.D. by Edinburgh, Physick returned to Philadelphia in the early 1790s and specialized in surgery. He was noted for his lithotomies (removal of stones), for the instrument he developed for tonsillectomies, and his introduction of buckskin sutures.

1805: First Boston medical library was founded.

1807: The University of Maryland medical school was organized as a private venture by a few physicians in Baltimore. It was the first of dozens of proprietary medical schools founded under state charters in the early 19th century. Training of physicians by apprenticeship continued and medical education remained brief and supplementary. By 1810 (after the closing of the independent Columbia College school), five American medical schools were functioning. The University of Pennsylvania (merged with the College of Philadelphia) predominated, and was attended by over 400 of the nation's 650 medical students.

1807: College of Physicians and Surgeons was chartered in New York City. It was absorbed in turn by Columbia University in 1891.

1809: Yale Medical School was founded.

1809: The first ovariotomy was performed by Dr. Ephraim McDowell in Danville, Kentucky.

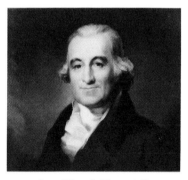

Caspar Wistar by Thomas Sully

1811: The first American textbook on anatomy was published. *A System of Anatomy* was a two-volume work by Dr. Caspar Wistar (1761-1818), professor at the University of Pennsylvania, and in whose honor wisteria was named.

1812: With the outbreak of the War of 1812, U.S. Navy surgeons went to sea with the fleet in growing numbers. A separate Medical Department had been established in 1811.

1812: First issue of the *New England Journal of Medicine* was published.

1812: *Medical Inquiries and Observations upon the Diseases of the Mind* by Dr. Benjamin Rush was first published.

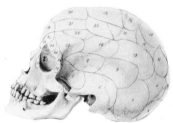

Phrenological Skull by T.R. Peale

1816: The first hospital-based ambulance service in the world was established at Bellevue Hospital, New York City.

1817: Medical school of Transylvania University opened in Lexington, Kentucky.

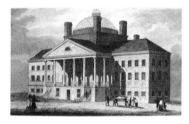

Massachusetts General Hospital

1818: Massachusetts General Hospital was erected from a design by Charles Bulfinch, architect. The hospital, founded in 1811, opened for patients in 1821.

1819: Medical College of Ohio was founded in Cincinnati.

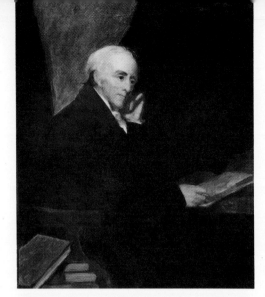

Benjamin Rush, M.D. Painting, c. 1804. [N.L.M.] Dr. Rush of Philadelphia, an early staff member of Pennsylvania Hospital, was educated in Edinburgh and London. *Below:* Print, 18th century. [L.C.P.] Rush had strong moral convictions and advocated diligent bleeding and purging (enemas) to drive ''vile humours'' from his patients' bodies.

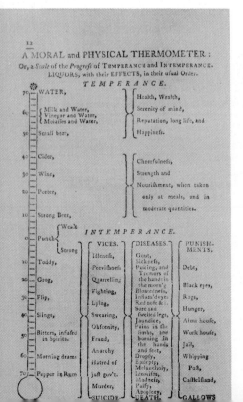

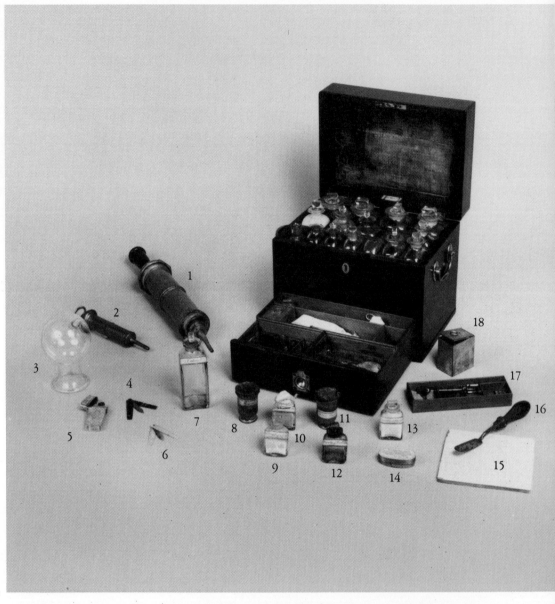

Above: Rush's Medical Chest. Wood and metal, 18th century. [P.C.P.S.] Includes:

1. pewter syringe for enemas
2. small pewter syringe
3. early American cupping glass
4. 18th century lancet
5. thumb lancet boxes
   A. tortoise
   B. mother-of-pearl
6. thumb lancets
7. empty calomel bottle
8. ointment jar with parchment cover—mercurial ointment
9. extract of lead
10. kid leather covered jar—Dover's Powder
11. ointment jar—yellow basilicon
12. parchment-covered ointment jar—Friar's balsam
13. emetic tartar
14. wooden box of Father Gill's pills
15. pill tile
16. spatula or spreader for compounding pills and plasters
17. wooden box containing apothecary scale (handheld) and weights
18. tin box for ointments

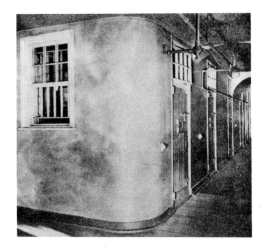

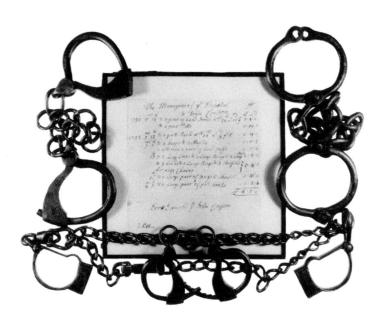

Above: Cells for Mental Patients. Below: Chains for Mental Patients. Photographs, 20th century. [P.H.] In the main, the mentally ill were treated simply by restraint and isolation behind bars, as at Pennsylvania Hospital on Pine Street.

MEDICAL INQUIRIES

AND

OBSERVATIONS,

UPON

THE DISEASES OF THE MIND.

BY BENJAMIN RUSH, M. D.
Professor of the Institutes and Practice of Medicine, and of Clinical Practice, in the University of Pennsylvania.

PHILADELPHIA:
PUBLISHED BY KIMBER & RICHARDSON,
NO. 237, MARKET STREET.
Merritt, Printer, No. 9, Watkin's Alley.
1812.

Left: Title Page. Print, 19th century. [P.H.] Rush was an early advocate of more humanitarian treatment for mental patients.

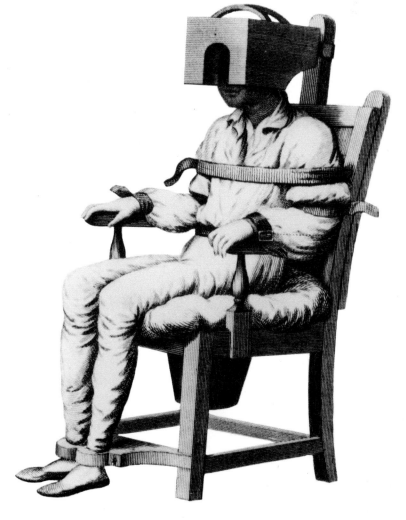

Right: The "Tranquilizing Chair." Engraving, 19th century. [N.L.M.] This alternative to cells and chains was developed by Dr. Benjamin Rush.

33

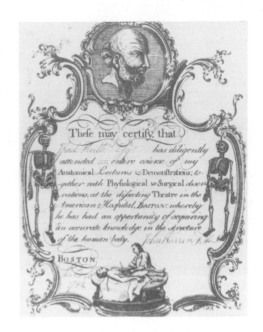

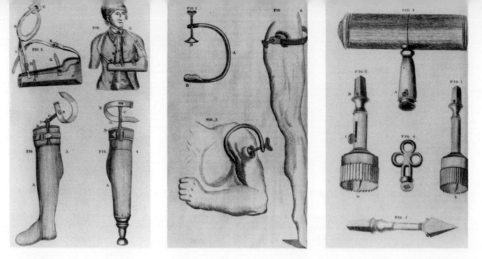

Above: Plates from Bell's *A System of Surgery*. Engravings, 18th century. [N.L.M.] Medical education, which was burgeoning throughout the new republic, was still largely derived from British and Scottish precepts and practice.

Above: Anatomical Lecture Certificate. Engraving by Paul Revere, 18th century. [M.7.] This was awarded by Dr. John Warren. *Right:* Massachusetts Medical College. Engraving, 19th century. [P.C.] It became the Harvard Medical School. *Below:* Benjamin Waterhouse. Painting by Gilbert Stuart, turn of the century. [N.L.M.]

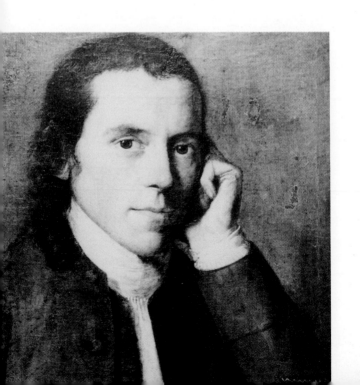

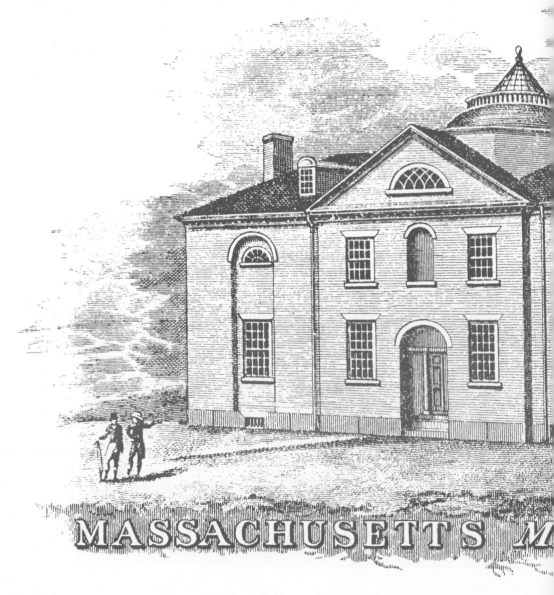

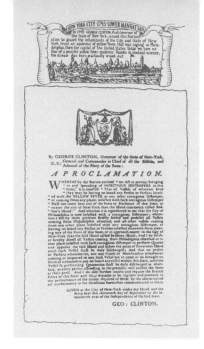

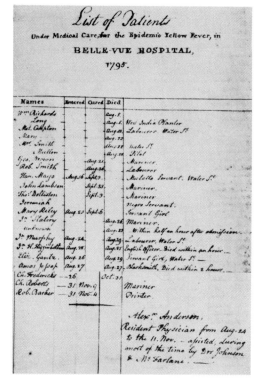

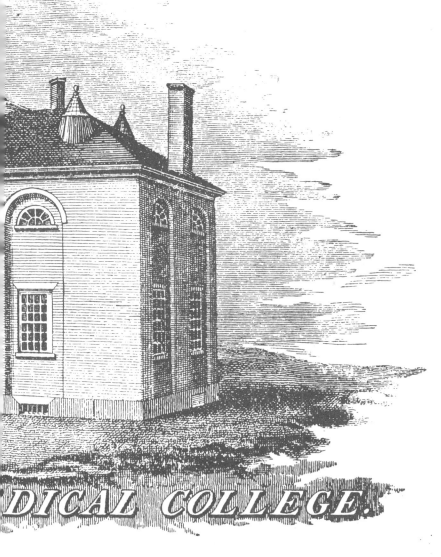

Above left: Quarantine Proclamation. Engraving, 18th century. [N.L.M.] The yellow fever epidemic that started in Philadelphia soon reached New York, where Governor Clinton issued this order in 1793. *Above:* Belle-Vue Hospital Patient List. 18th century. [N.Y.A.M.] Dr. Alexander Anderson made this list of yellow fever patients admitted to the hospital in 1795. *Below:* New York Hospital. Engraving, 19th century. [N.L.M.] By 1810, New York Hospital was one of the nation's leading institutions.

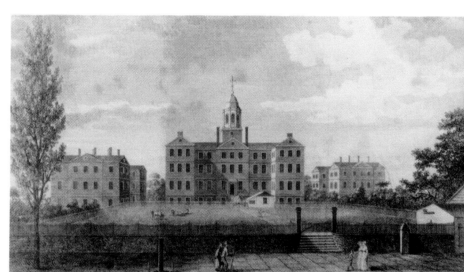

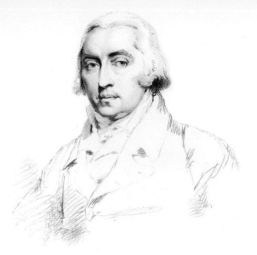

Above: Dr. Philip Syng Physick. Engraving, 19th century. [N.L.M.] Physick, 1768–1837, was a remarkably skilled and innovative surgeon. He was among the first to remove cataracts, correct harelips and, in 1812, is known to have employed a stomach pump to save a child who had swallowed poison. *Below:* Title Page of Physick's Thesis on Apoplexia. 18th century. [N.L.M.]

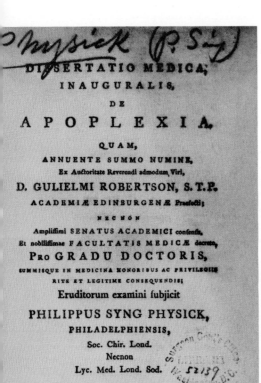

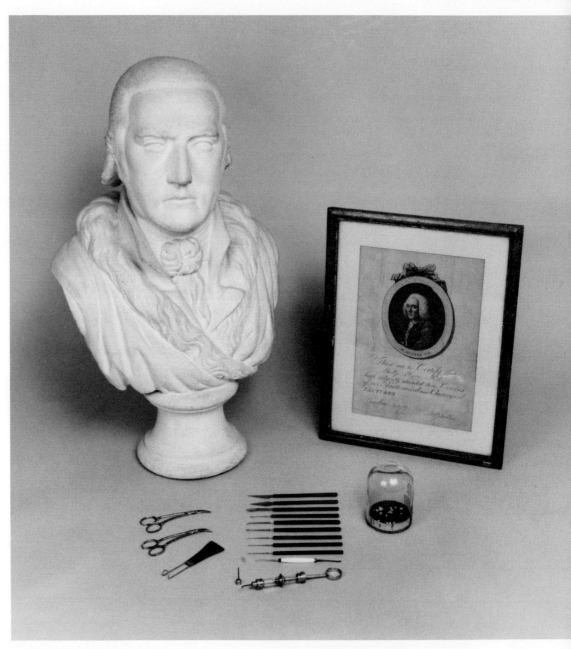

Above: Bust (marble, 19th century); Diploma, Instruments (mixed materials). [P.C.P.S.] Among Physick's most famous operations was the removal, in 1831, of a stone from the bladder of Chief Justice John Marshall, then in his 76th year.

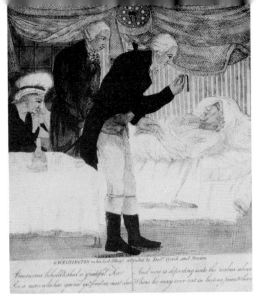

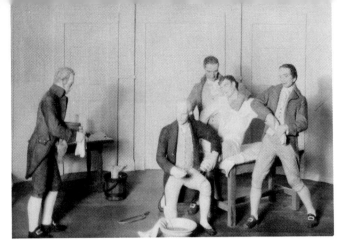

Above: Death of George Washington. Print, 19th century. [N.A.] The President is being attended by Doctors Craik and Brown. The caption reads: "Americans behold and shed a grateful Tear; For a man who has gained you freedom most dear. And now is departing unto the realms above; where he may ever rest in lasting peace and love." *Above right:* Physick Operating. Diorama. (J.J.) Physick deservedly prospered; toward the end of his life he earned $20,000 a year and left an estate of more than half a million dollars.

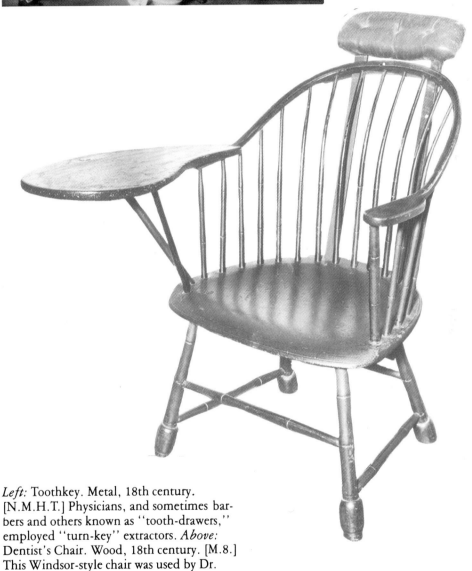

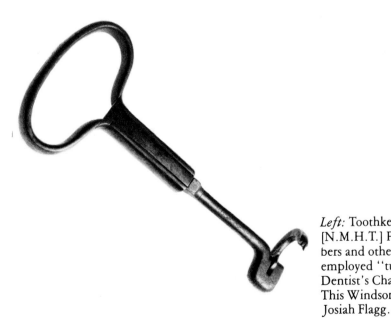

Left: Toothkey. Metal, 18th century. [N.M.H.T.] Physicians, and sometimes barbers and others known as "tooth-drawers," employed "turn-key" extractors. *Above:* Dentist's Chair. Wood, 18th century. [M.8.] This Windsor-style chair was used by Dr. Josiah Flagg.

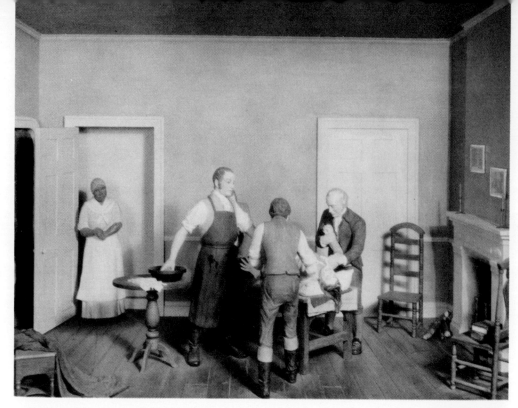

Right: Diorama from Century of Progress Exhibit, Chicago, 1933, Depicting McDowell's Milestone Operation. [J.J.]
Below: Ephraim McDowell, M.D., Father of Abdominal Surgery. Engraving, 19th century. [A.M.A.] Americans were moving West, often across the Appalachian Trail to Danville, Ky., McDowell's home.

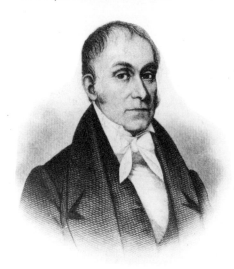

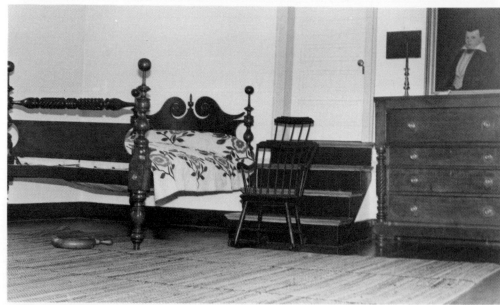

Left: McDowell's Federal-style House as It Looks Today. Photograph, 20th century. [E.M.H.] In it were his office and pharmacy. Although the house was not grand, it suggests he had an established practice. *Above:* Restored Room in McDowell's House. Photograph, 20th century. [E.M.H.] Here McDowell surgically removed a 20-pound ovarian tumor from his 45-year-old patient. Lacking any anesthetic, Mrs. Crawford chanted hymns and psalms to fight the pain. Five days later, McDowell found her "up and making her bed." She returned home in good health and lived to be 78.

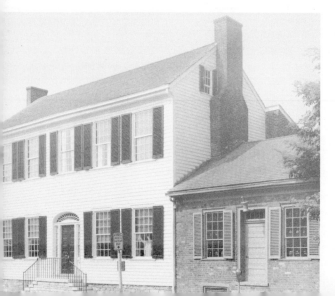

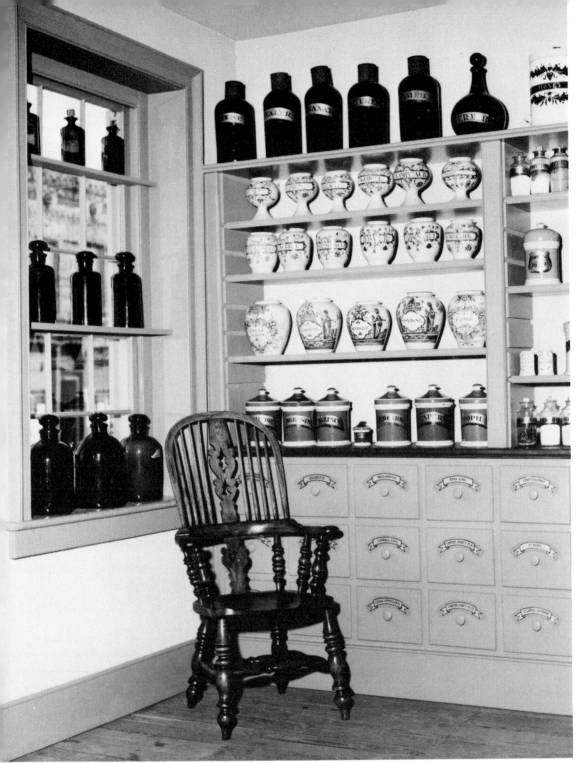

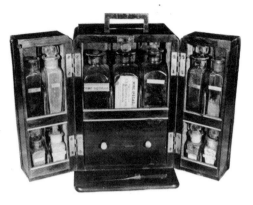

Above: McDowell's Medicine Case. Mixed materials. Photograph, 20th century. [E.M.H.]
Left: McDowell's Apothecary Shop. Photograph, 20th century. [E.M.H.]
McDowell provided pharmaceutical as well as medical services to his patients.

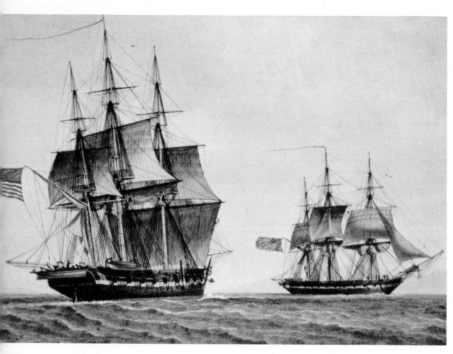

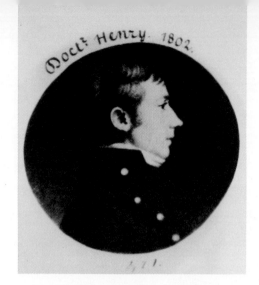

Dr. Isaac Henry. Painting, c. 1802. [U.S.D.N.] Dr. Henry, a naval surgeon, served on the U.S.S. *Constellation* during the war with England.

Above: U.S. Navy Frigates. Painting, 19th century. [P.C.] As America's maritime trade expanded in the early 19th century, so did her navy. In 1798 and 1799, Congress passed laws requiring a monthly assessment of 20 cents from U.S. Navy and merchant seamen. Under the "Navy Pension Fund" all sick and disabled "officers, seamen and marines" were to be cared for in hospitals supported in part by the assessment. In 1811, legislation established a separate Medical Department of the Navy. *Right:* 18th Century Pharmacy. Photograph. [A.P.A.] Ships' captains and surgeons secured drugs and medicinal spirits from coastal pharmacies like this restored apothecary shop.

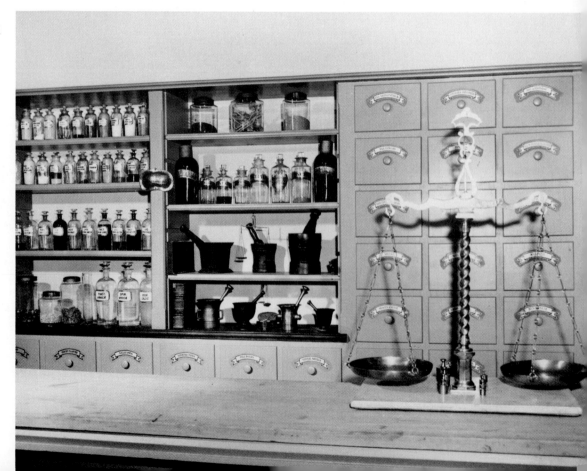

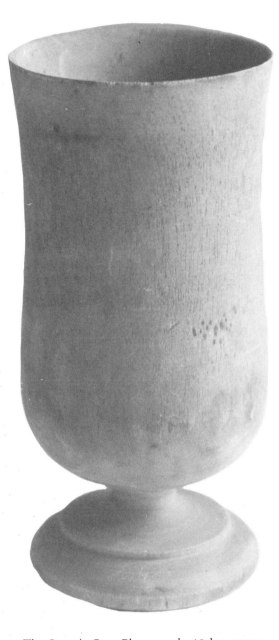

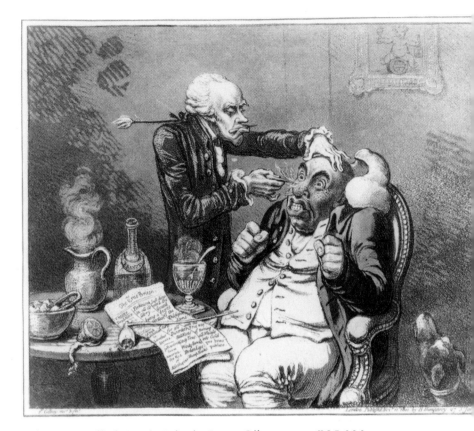

Above: A Medical Quack. Print by James Gilray, 1801. [N.L.M.] Despite satirical drawings, such as this one which appeared in London, metallic tractors were popular there and in America. *Below:* Perkins' Tractors. Photograph, metal, 19th century. [H.M.S.] Invented by Dr. Elisha Perkins of Connecticut, the magnetic tractors were supposed to effect miraculous cures by merely being drawn across the skin.

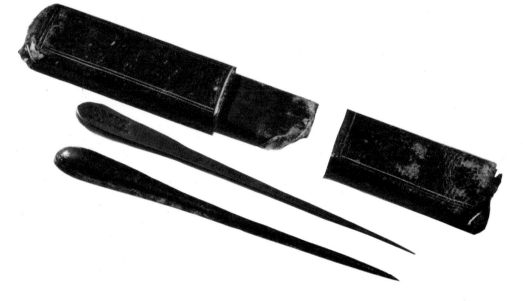

The Quassia Cup. Photograph, 19th century. [E.L.] An early and popular nostrum. The cup, made from the wood of a South American tree, was filled with boiling water, and the resulting infusion was administered as a bitter tonic to cure some 27 diseases—from fevers to worms to malignancies. Introduced in the 1750s, it was still being sold in the late 19th century.

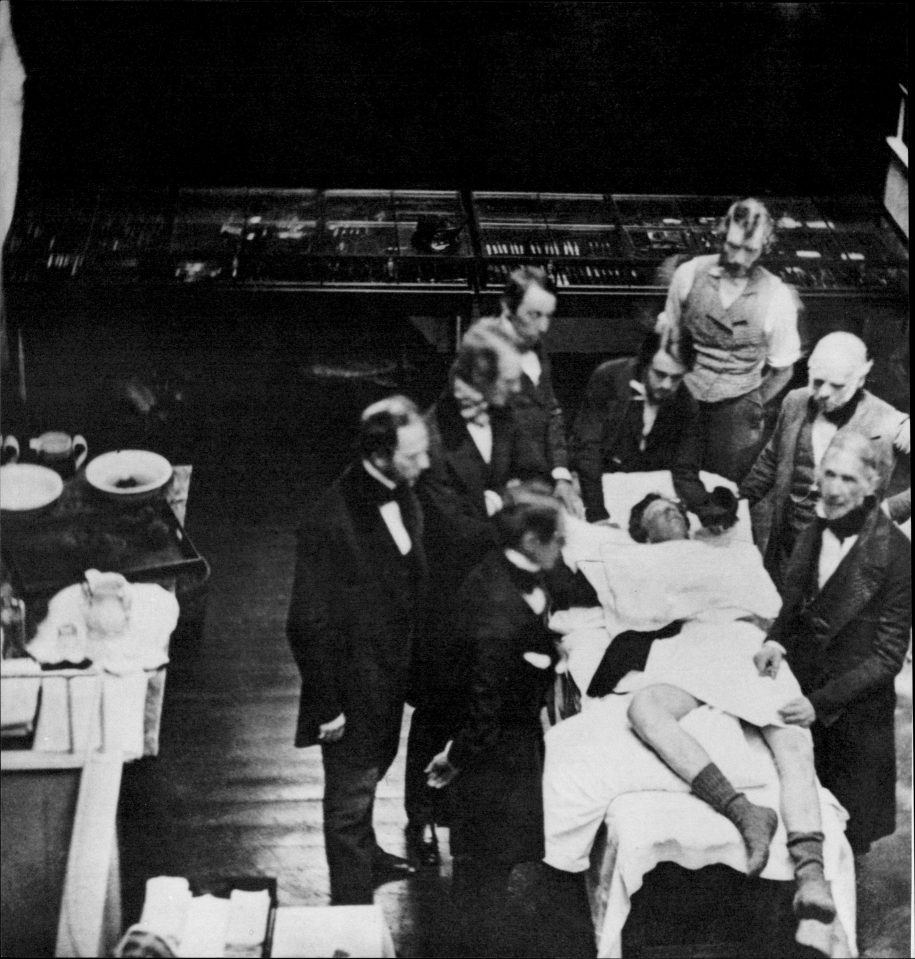

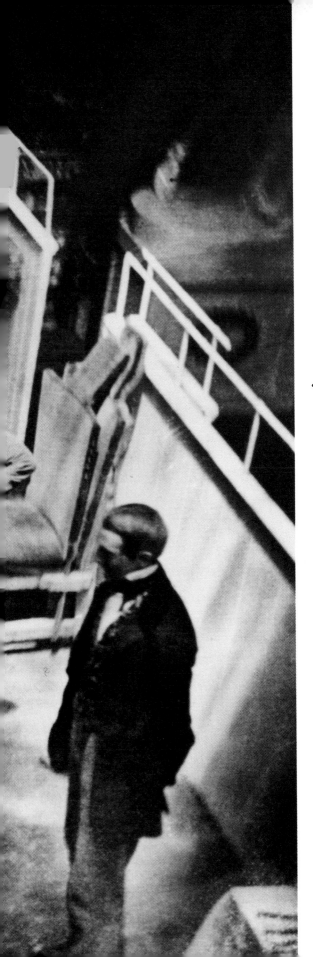

CHAPTER THREE

1820-1859

Dr. John Richmond, one of many daring and enterprising physicians of the Old West, performed the first recorded cesarian section west of the Alleghenies in Newton, Ohio in 1827. He later recalled: "I had no recourse to cordials, for these could not be obtained. I was seven miles from home, and had but few medicines with me. After doing all in my power for her preservation, and feeling myself entirely in the dark as to her situation, and finding that whatever was done, must be done soon, and feeling a deep and solemn sense of my responsibility, with only a case of common pocket instruments, about one o'clock at night, I commenced the cesarian section . . . I was convinced that the patient must die, or the operation be performed. The patient never complained of pain during the whole course of the cure. She commenced work in twenty-four days from the operation."

As Americans moved West in increasing numbers in the first half of the 19th century, physicians, lured by the same prospect of adventure, glory and wealth, followed suit. The reality, however, showed a pioneer physician's life to be one of peril, toil and privation. Conditions were primitive, and because manufactured medicines were often unavailable, doctors frequently concocted their own. Thus the "primitive" medicine of the frontier became the foundation on which a modern science was building.

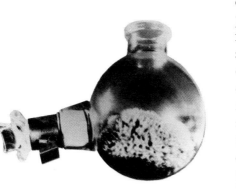

Left: Operating Room of the Massachusetts General Hospital, Boston. Daguerreotype, 19th century. [M.G.H.] This was a reenactment of the initial demonstration of ether anesthesia on October 16, 1846. *Above:* Morton-Gould Ether Inhaler, 1847 Patent Model, Metal. [M.G.H.]

1820: Maine became 23rd state
9,638,000 inhabitants: 2,000,000 in West
Missouri Compromise
Monroe reelected President
1821: Missouri became 24th state
1823: Monroe Doctrine announced
1824-25: John Quincy Adams declared President by House of Representatives
1826: New parties, Democratic Republicans and National Republicans
Erie Canal opened
1826: July 4, Thomas Jefferson, John Adams died
1827-38: Irish and German migration to U.S.
1828: Andrew Jackson elected President
Construction of Baltimore & Ohio RR started
1829: Jackson inaugurated
1830: 12,866,020 inhabitants reported
1831: Nat Turner led slave rebellion
1832: Jackson reelected President
Black Hawk War
1833: American Anti-Slavery Society formed
1834-39: Davenport invented electric motor
1835: Colt patented the revolver
1836: Arkansas became 25th state
Battles of the Alamo and San Jacinto
1837: Michigan became 26th state
U.S. recognized Texas

1820

1830

1820: The first United States Pharmacopoeia was issued.

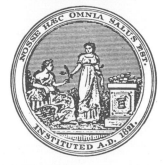

Seal of The Philadelphia College of Pharmacy

1821: The nation's first school of pharmacy was formed, the Philadelphia College of Pharmacy and Science.

1821: Massachusetts General Hospital opened in Boston. A pioneering institution, the 93-bed hospital had special training for medical students, and paying patients as well as paupers.

1822: A classic study of gastric physiology began with the shooting in northern Michigan of a French-Canadian trapper, who was treated by an army surgeon at Fort Michilimackinac. The patient lived—with a permanently unhealed exterior opening giving access to his stomach. The physician, William Beaumont (1785-1853), took advantage of this rare opportunity to undertake experiments on the digestive process.

1825: *American Journal of Pharmacy* began publication.

1831: Chloroform was discovered. A few months before its nearly simultaneous discovery in France and Germany, chloroform was discovered by Samuel Guthrie (1782-1848), a Massachusetts-born physician. For years the substance he found was regarded only as a chemical curiosity and intoxicant. Not until 1847 were its anesthetic qualities recognized and put to use in Scotland.

1832: A cholera epidemic killed 6,000 in New Orleans, tens of thousands more in other American and Canadian cities. Other cholera epidemics in 1849, 1866 and 1873 took heavy tolls in the East and spread up the Mississippi river valley into the Midwest. The disease was carried by passengers of riverboats and wagon trains. Red pepper and whiskey were given to the dying.

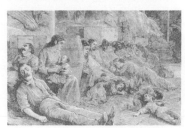

Interior of a Riverboat, a Cholera Breeding Ground

1832: Boston Lying-In Hospital was established.

1839: A flexible-tube stethoscope was invented by C.W. Pennock of Philadelphia. Diagnosis was made easier by replacement of the rigid, awkward wooden stethoscope devised by Rene Laennec of France at the beginning of the century.

1839: The world's first dental school, the Baltimore College of Dental Surgery, was founded. The following year the American Society of Dental Surgeons was established.

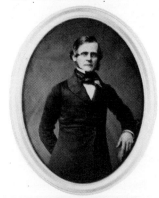

Dr. Thomas Story Kirkbride, a Philadephia Pioneer Reformer of Mental Institutions

1841: Dorothea Dix (1802-1887), visited a Massachusetts jail and was horrified at indiscriminate mixing of criminals and the imprisoned insane. The following year Dix wrote a famous appeal to the state legislature demanding humane specialized care for the mentally ill. Her successful crusade led to the founding of many state hospitals for the insane.

1842: Ether was probably first used as a general anesthetic by Dr. Crawford Long of Georgia. Ether, chloroform and nitrous oxide, the three basic anesthetics, had been known for years but never applied to medicine. Long (1815-1878), a physician in Jefferson, Georgia, performed three small operations using sulfuric ether, but he did not publicize his success until anesthesia had been generally recognized.

1844: A Connecticut dentist, Dr. Horace Wells (1815-1848), demonstrated the analgesic properties of nitrous oxide by having one of his own teeth extracted while under its influence. Wells administered "laughing gas" successfully to several of his own patients, but failed to convince Dr. John C. Warren's medical class at Harvard of the value of his discovery.

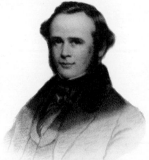

Dr. Horace Wells

1844: The American Psychiatric Association was founded.

44

1840: 17,069,456 inhabitants reported
William Henry Harrison elected President

1841: First wagon train to California
Harrison died in office; John Tyler succeeded

1844: James K. Polk elected President
Morse sent message over first telegraph

1845: Florida became 27th state
Texas became 28th state
U.S. Naval Academy opened

1846: Iowa became 29th state

1846-48: War with Mexico

1848: Wisconsin became 30th state
Gold discovered in California
Zachary Taylor elected President

1850: 23,261,000 inhabitants; 35.9% over 1840
California admitted as 31st state
Taylor died; Millard Fillmore succeeded to Presidency

1851: 221,253 Irish immigrants arrived in U.S.

1852: Franklin Pierce, Democrat, elected President
Stowe's *Uncle Tom's Cabin* published

1853-56: Crimean War

1854: Republican Party formed

1856: John C. Fremont, first Republican
candidate, defeated by Buchanan for Presidency

1857: Supreme Court announced Dred Scott decision

1858: Minnesota became 32nd state
Lincoln and Douglas debated in Illinois

1859: Darwin's *Origin of Species* published
Oregon became 33rd state
Supreme Court upheld Fugitive
Slave Act

1840   1850   1859

1846: Surgery without pain—sulfuric ether used as a general anesthetic—was first publicly demonstrated at the Massachusetts General Hospital. Dr. William T.G. Morton (1819-1868), a dentist, succeeded in convincing his medical colleagues. News of the process, named "anesthesia" by Oliver Wendell Holmes, spread quickly across North America and to Europe.

1847: Oliver Wendell Holmes—physician, poet, essayist and teacher—became dean of Harvard Medical School.

1847: New York Academy of Medicine was founded.

1847: American Medical Association was founded. State and local medical societies joined to form a national organization dedicated to improving professional education and ethics, as well as public health.

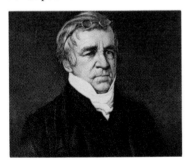

Dr. Nathaniel Chapman,
First A.M.A. President

1848: A college for midwives was established in Boston by Dr. Samuel Gregory. It was an attempt to encourage trained female midwives to reenter the field that male physicians had gradually monopolized since the 1780s.

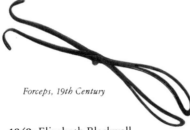

Forceps, 19th Century

1849: Elizabeth Blackwell (1821-1910), became the first woman in the United States to receive a medical degree. Born in England, Blackwell graduated from Geneva Medical College, New York.

1850: University of Michigan Medical School was founded.

1851: The Female Medical College of Pennsylvania, the first woman's medical college in the world, opened in Philadelphia. In 1867 it was renamed The Woman's Medical College of Pennsylvania.

1852: The American Pharmaceutical Association was launched by 20 delegates meeting in the hall of the Philadelphia College of Pharmacy and Science.

1855: Woman's Hospital was founded in New York City by Dr. J. Marion Sims (1813-1883). Sims laid the basis for gynecology as a specialty. He introduced the vaginal speculum, and later, (1866), wrote the important *Clinical Notes on Uterine Surgery*.

1855: The binaural stethoscope was invented by Dr. George P. Cammann of New York.

1855: The Jews' Hospital opened on West 28th Street in New York City. Open to all patients, the hospital changed its name to Mount Sinai in 1866.

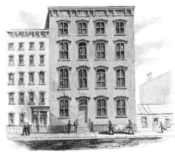

Mount Sinai Hospital, New York City

1857: New York Infirmary for Women and Children was founded. Founders were Dr. Elizabeth Blackwell, her sister Dr. Emily Blackwell (1826-1910), and Polish-born Dr. Maria Elizabeth Zakrzewska (1829-1902). In 1868 the hospital was expanded to include a Women's College for the training of doctors.

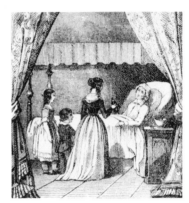

Detail from Mid-19th Century
Drug Advertisement

1857: William Richard Warner opened a drugstore and began manufacturing pharmaceutical products in Philadelphia. Warner was one of the first to mask the bitter taste of medication by coating pills with sugar.

1858: The pharmaceutical company of E.R. Squibb was founded.

1859: The Chicago Medical College at Lind University (later Northwestern) was founded. This school was one of the first to reform its standards of medical education. For 50 years, almost any student who could pay had been admitted and graduated as a physician after lectures lasting no more than 14 weeks. Lind raised entrance requirements and lengthened the course. Ten years later, Harvard followed suit.

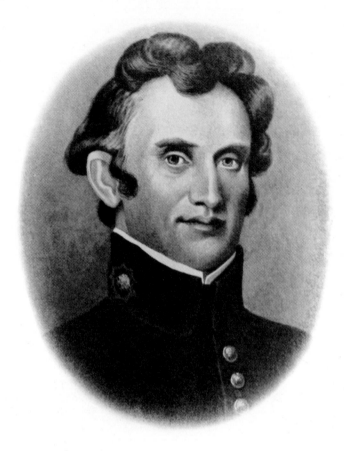

Left: Dr. William Beaumont, (1785-1853). Print, 19th century. *Below:* Beaumont's License to Practice Medicine. Print, 1812. [N.L.M.]

BY THE THIRD MEDICAL SOCIETY
OF THE STATE OF VERMONT,
AS BY LAW ESTABLISHED.

William Beaumont having presented himself to this Society for examination Anatomy of the Human Body, and the Theory and Practice of Physic and Surgery being approved by our Censors, the society willingly recommend him to the world as cious and safe practitioner in the different avocations of the Medical Profession. timony whereof we have hereunto prefixed the signature of our President and Seal of ciety, at the Medical Hall in Burlington, the 2d. Tuesday of *June* A. D

Cassius F. Pomeroy, Secretary.   Jno. Pomeroy, Pre

Below: Regulations of the Hartford Medical Society together with Fee Table. Print, September 15, 1846. [H.M.S.] The preamble states that, despite the increase of living expenses, the new table of fees is "with some slight alterations identical with the former one" — in effect since 1813. House calls were $1.00, except "from 11 P.M. to sunrise," when they were $2.00.

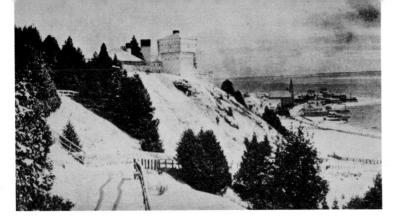

Left: Fort Michilimackinac. Photograph, 20th century. [N.Y.A.M.] It was here that Beaumont began his classic study of gastric physiology. Midwinter scene shows blockhouse surgeons' quarters and hospital. *Below left:* View of St. Louis. Print, 1840-46. [C.H.S.] By the late 1840s, St. Louis, as the gateway to the West, was a fast-growing city. *Below right:* First hospital in St. Louis. Photograph, 20th century. [M.10.] In 1828 this cabin became the city's first hospital.

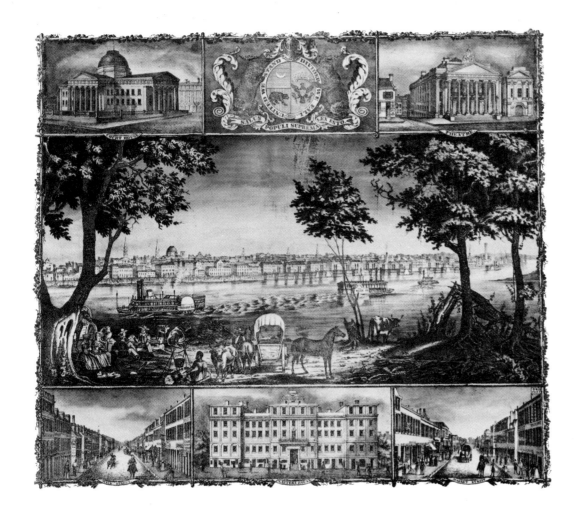

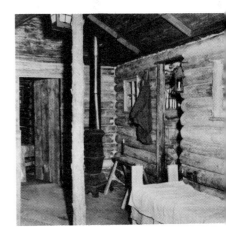

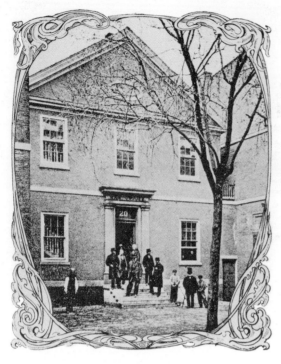

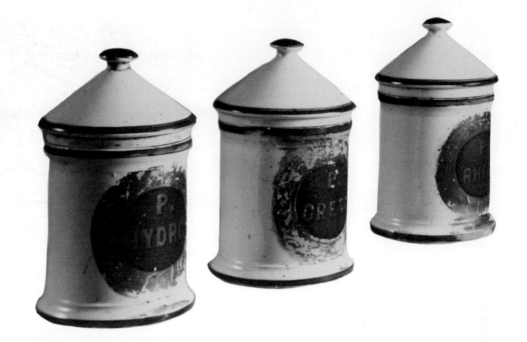

Above: First home of the Philadelphia College of Pharmacy and Science. Daguerrotype, 19th century. [P.C.P.] *Right:* Apothecary Jars. Porcelain, mid 19th century. [E.L.] These jars were used by a Little Rock, Arkansas doctor.

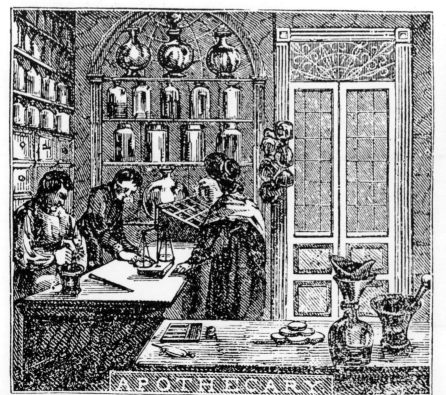

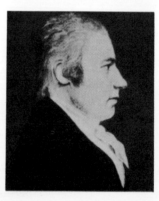 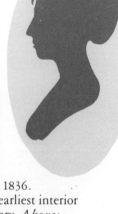

Left: Apothecary Shop. Print, 1836. [S.P.U.W.] This is one of the earliest interior views of an American apothecary. *Above:* Charles Marshall. Painting, 19th century. [P.C.P.] Marshall was the first president of the Philadelphia College of Pharmacy and Science. Elizabeth Marshall. Silhouette, 19th century. [P.C.P.] Marshall's daughter was one of the first women to have practiced pharmacy in this country.

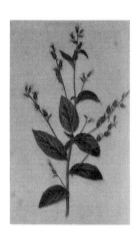
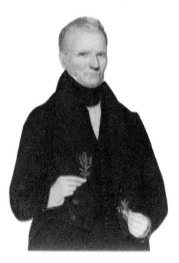

Above left: Lobelia. Print, 19th century. [N.L.M.] This herb was prescribed for all complaints known to man, from dyspepsia and croup to cancer and tuberculosis. *Above right:* Samuel Thomson. Painting, 19th century. [N.L.M.] In 1822, Thomson, a self-proclaimed herb-and-root doctor, published his *New Guide to Health; or, Botanic Family Physician.* By 1830 he claimed over three million adherents. *Below:* Engraving, 19th century. [N.L.M.] This "Thomsonian" ad appeared in 1835.

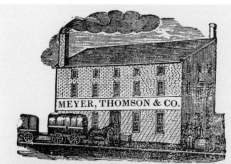

WHOLESALE & RETAIL
THOMSONIAN
BOTANIC MEDICINE STORE.

The subscribers have the largest and most valuable collection of

BOTANIC MEDICINES

in the United States, comprising all the compounds and crude articles recommended by Dr. Samuel Thomson, part of which is as follows:

African Cayenne	Lobelia,—do. Seed
Balmony	Nerve Ointment
Barberry	Nerve Powder
Butter Nut Syrup	Pond Lily
Cancer Plaster	Poplar Bark. coarse and fine
Clivers	Prickly Ash
Composition	Raspberry Leaves
Conserve of Hollyhock	Slippery Elm
Cough Powder	Woman's Friend or Females'
Ginger	Bitters
Golden Seal	Unicorn Root
Gum Myrrh	Wake Robin. &c. &c. &c.

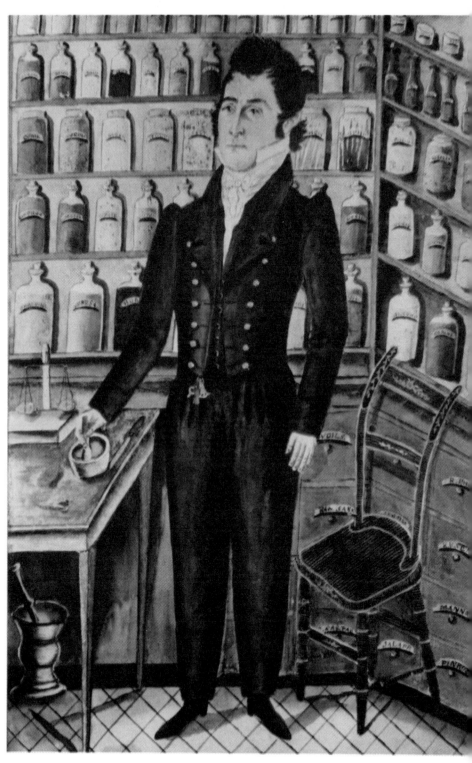

Above: Dr. Christian Bucher. Painting, c. 1840. [P.C.] Dr. Bucher was an established physician and pharmacist of Schaefferstown, Pa.

Right: Frontier Doctor. Engraving, 19th century. [L.C.] Frontier doctors might ride 60 miles to make a call, and often slept on the trail. *Below:* Saddlebag with Drugs. 19th century. [A.H.S.] The drugs carried by this frontier practitioner, a Georgian, included Calomel, a mercury-based cathartic; Ipecac, an emetic (to induce vomiting); Morphine, Quinine, and Camphor. *Bottom:* Leather Saddlebags. 19th century. [M.12.] These saddlebags were used by Dr. Marcus Whitman, the first Missionary physician in the Oregon Territory.

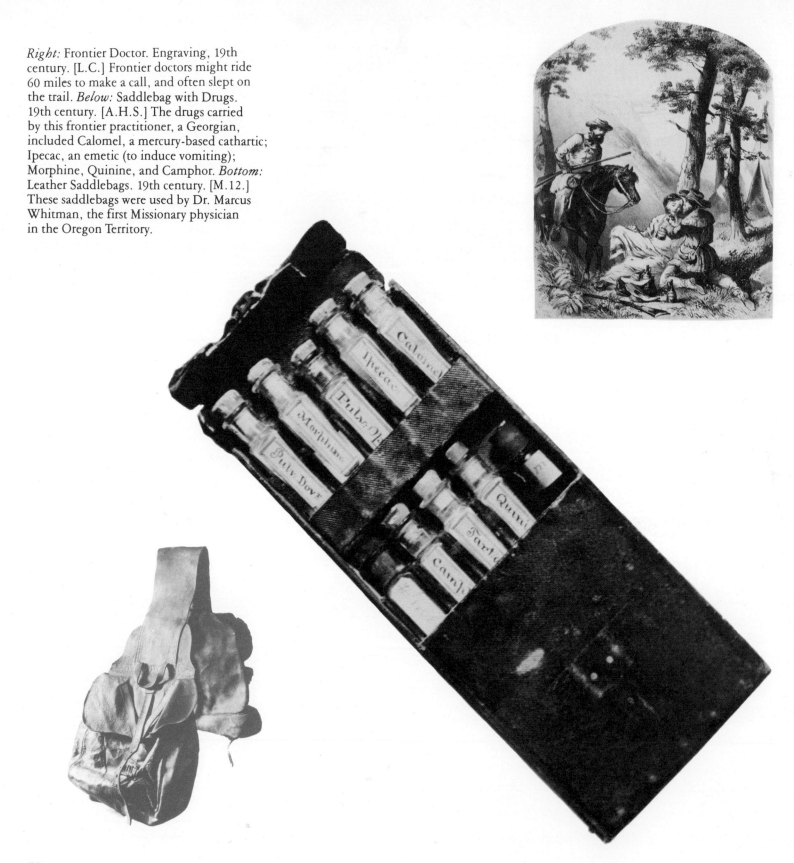

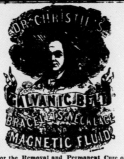

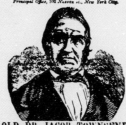

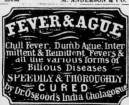

Left: Mobile Advertiser. Newspaper, July 6, 1849. [H.M.P.S.] Medical nostrums, as proclaimed in this Alabama weekly newspaper, purported to cure anything—for a price. *Below:* A Midwife's Advertisement. *Mobile Advertiser*, July 6, 1849.

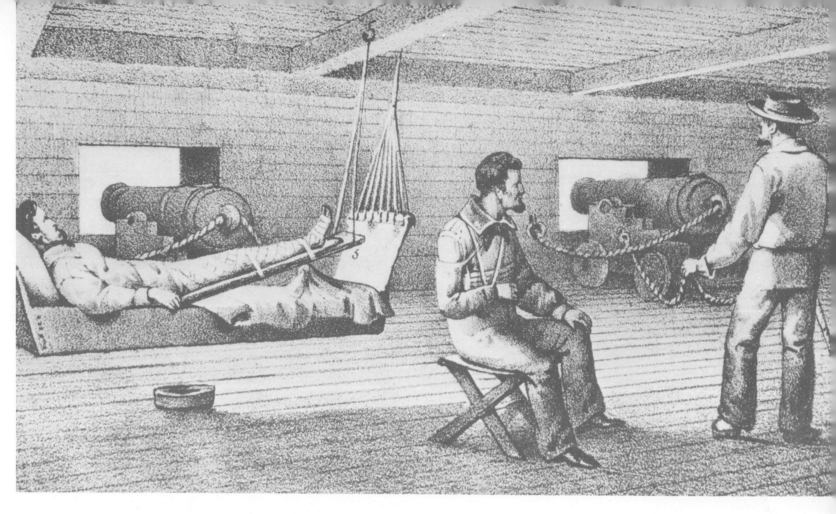

Above: Injured Bluejackets Aboard a U.S. Navy Sailing Vessel. Engraving, c. 1845. [P.C.] By the 1840s, American flagships plied all the oceans and seas of the world and Naval Surgeons were aboard. *Below right:* Surgeon Elisha Kent Kane. Painting, 19th century. [U.S.N.A.] *Below left:* U.S. Marine Hospital. Watercolor, 1830. [N.L.M.] This naval hospital was at Chelsea, Mass., near the busy port of Boston.

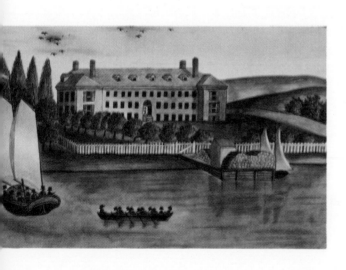

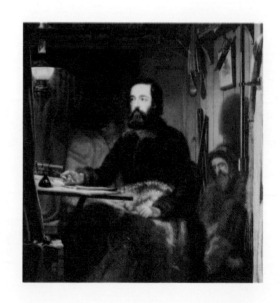

52

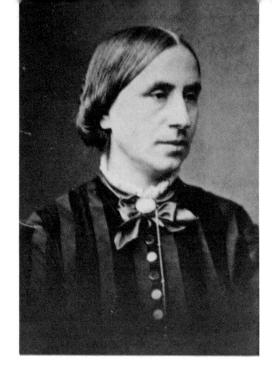

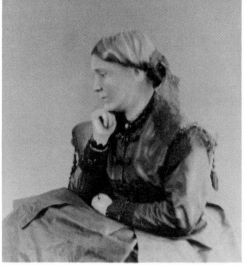

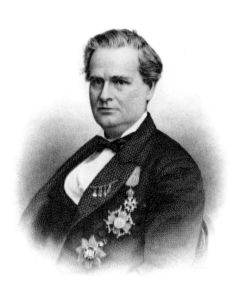

Above: Dr. Maria Zakrzewska. Daguerreotype, 19th century. [N.Y.A.M.] Born in Poland, Dr. Zakrzewska was instrumental in the founding of the New York Infirmary for Women and Children (1857), and Boston's New England Hospital for Women & Children (1859). *Center:* Elizabeth Blackwell, M.D. Daguerreotype, 19th century. [N.L.M.] *Above right:* Dr. J. Marion Sims. Engraving, 19th century. [N.L.M.] *Right:* Dr. Sims, Surgeon of the Diseases of Women. Diorama, 20th century. [J.J.] He is seen holding the speculum which he devised.

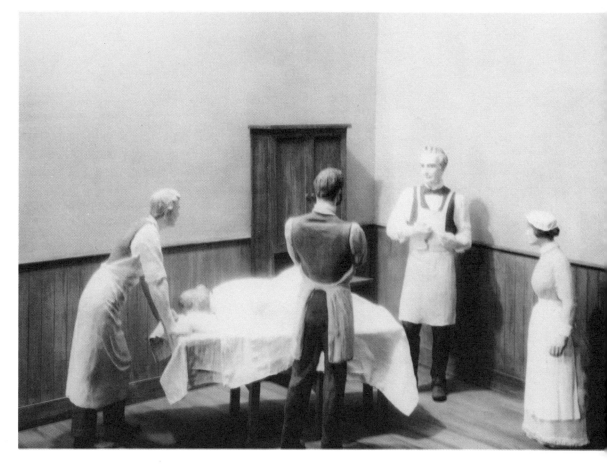

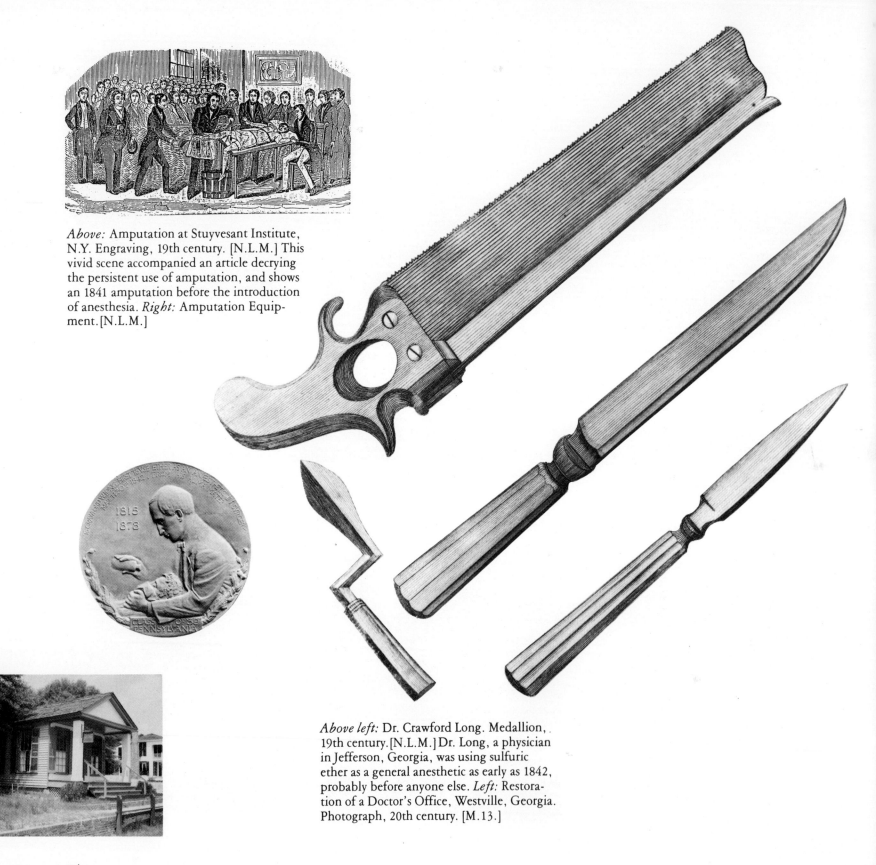

Above: Amputation at Stuyvesant Institute, N.Y. Engraving, 19th century. [N.L.M.] This vivid scene accompanied an article decrying the persistent use of amputation, and shows an 1841 amputation before the introduction of anesthesia. *Right:* Amputation Equipment. [N.L.M.]

Above left: Dr. Crawford Long. Medallion, 19th century. [N.L.M.] Dr. Long, a physician in Jefferson, Georgia, was using sulfuric ether as a general anesthetic as early as 1842, probably before anyone else. *Left:* Restoration of a Doctor's Office, Westville, Georgia. Photograph, 20th century. [M.13.]

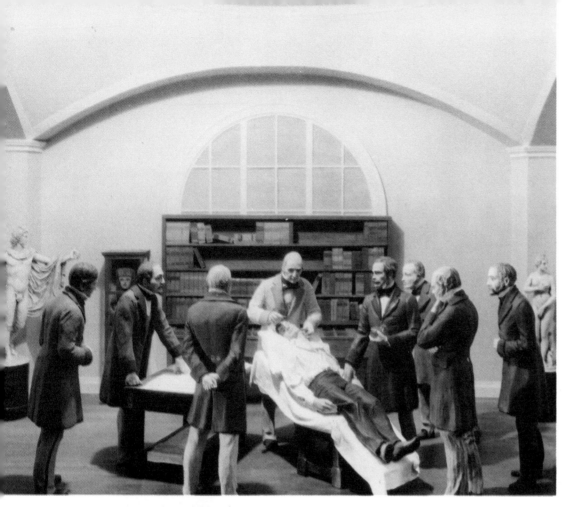

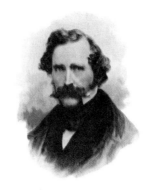

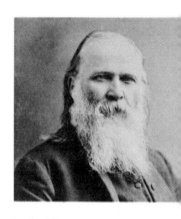

Left: Dr. William T.G. Morton in the First Public Demonstration of the Anesthetic Effects of Ether; Dr. John Collins Warren Operating. Diorama, 20th century. [J.J.] *Above left:* William Morton. Painting, 19th century.[N.L.M.] Morton was instructed in dental techniques by Horace Wells. *Above right:* Dr. W.H. Atkinson. Photograph, 19th century. [M.14.] First president of the American Dental Association, founded in 1859.

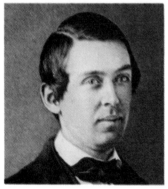

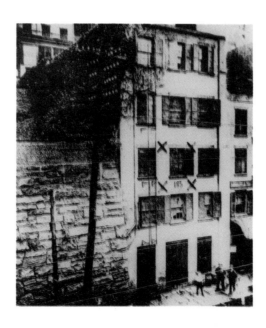

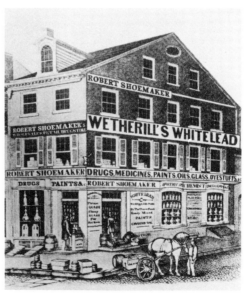

Above: Dr. Edward Robinson Squibb. Daguerreotype by Matthew Brady, 19th century. [E.R.S.] Dr. Squibb served as a naval surgeon and formed a pharmaceutical house in 1858. *Right:* Squibb's Brooklyn Plant. Daguerreotype, 19th century. [E.R.S.] *Far right:* Robert Shoemaker's Drugstore. Daguerreotype, c. 1850. [S.P.U.W.]

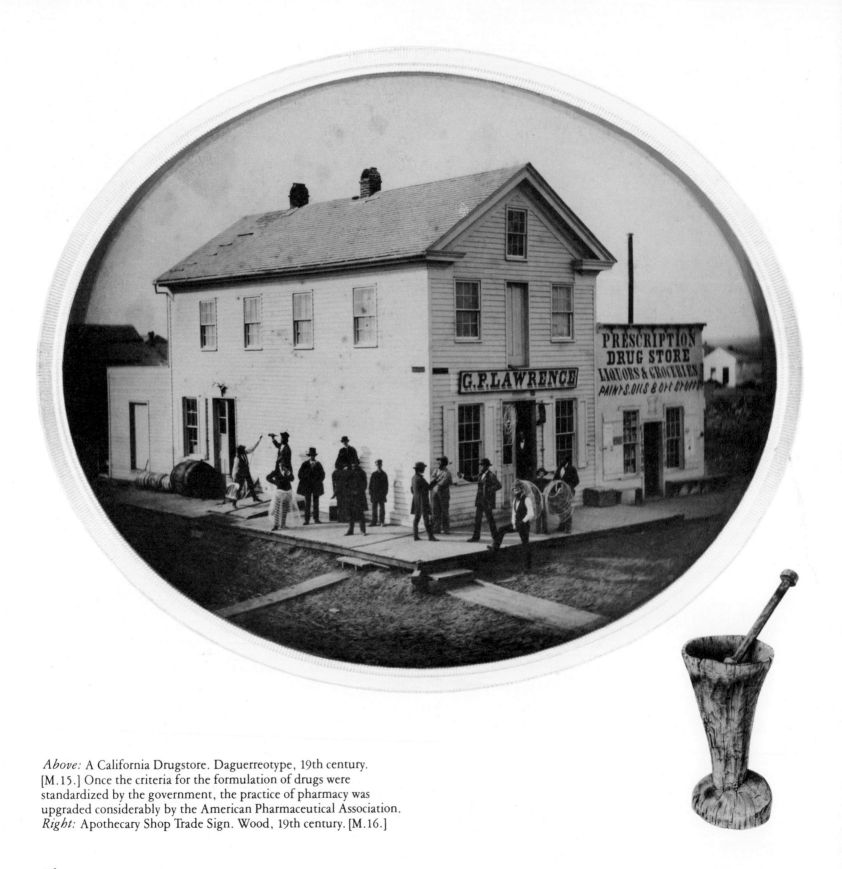

Above: A California Drugstore. Daguerreotype, 19th century.
[M.15.] Once the criteria for the formulation of drugs were
standardized by the government, the practice of pharmacy was
upgraded considerably by the American Pharmaceutical Association.
Right: Apothecary Shop Trade Sign. Wood, 19th century. [M.16.]

56

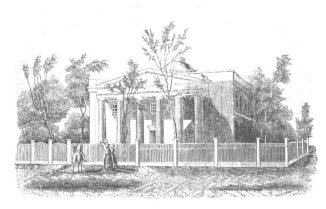

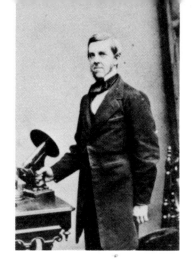

Above: Medical College of Georgia. Engraving, c. 1848. [P.C.] By mid-century, institutions of medical training were spreading across the country. A dominant figure in medical education at the time was, *Above right:* Dr. Oliver Wendell Holmes. Daguerreotype, c. 1855. [P.C.]

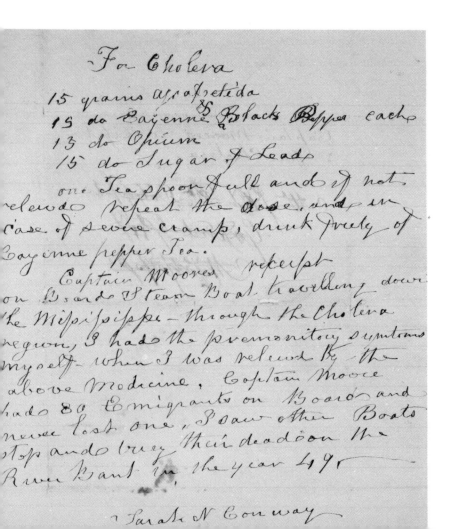

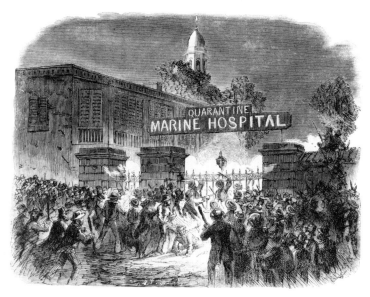

Left: Cholera Antidote Recipe. Pen and ink, 19th century. [H.M.P.S.] During the 1849 cholera epidemic, Sarah Conway of Mobile recorded in her diary this recipe given her by Capt. Moore, a Mississippi steamboat captain. *Above:* Quarantine Riot. Engraving, 1858. [L.C.] *Harper's Weekly* described this riot on Staten Island, New York, when townspeople sought to burn down a "plague house."

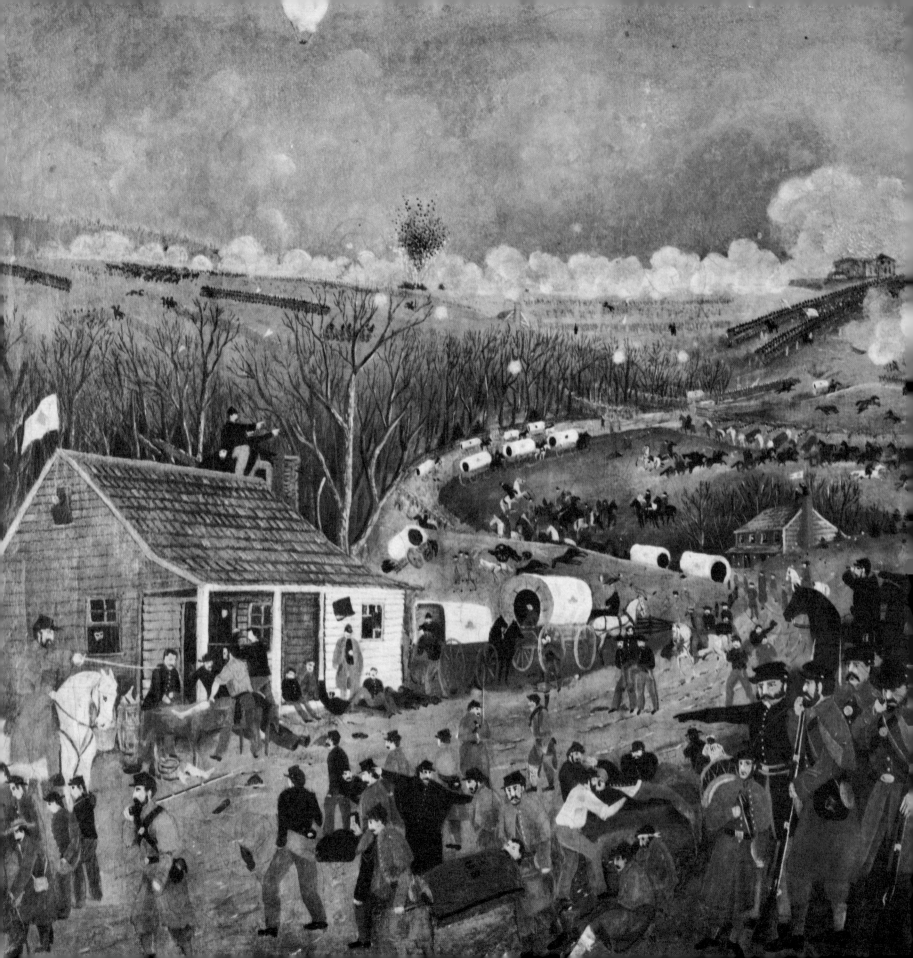

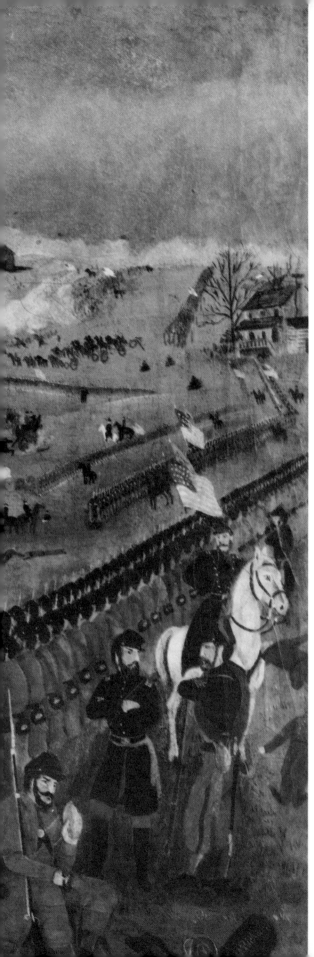

CHAPTER FOUR

1860-1879

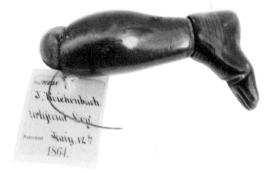

Emma French-Sackett, one of countless women from both North and South who volunteered to serve as nurses in the Civil War, wrote this poignant account of her experience: "...although sad the office we performed, our hearts were filled with pleasure in the work we were doing. It was ours to minister to the wants of mind and body; and when the poor soldier boy had breathed his last, to write to his parents, wife or sister, telling of his last hours, and giving the messages for loved ones at home... those to whom I ministered seemed to me more like brothers than strangers."

When the North and South became engulfed in a civil war, women from around the country and all walks of life answered a compelling need to contribute their services, and in doing so defied the traditional strictures that had regulated their lives. Despite the government's reticence and skepticism, women in the North managed to organize and coordinate their efforts under the aegis of the United States Sanitary Commission. In the South, women's contributions were no less important.

The War brought to the forefront the unrecognized professional talents of such remarkable and valiant women as Clara Barton and Dr. Mary Edwards Walker. Gradually the medical world, a predominantly masculine one, began to take heed of women's potential in medicine, and particularly in the field of nursing, which was yet to be established.

Left: Field Hospital at Battle of Fredericksburg. Painting, 19th century. [P.C.] *Above:* Prosthetic Patented Wooden Leg, 1864. [N.M.H.T.]

1861: Kansas became 33rd state
Confederate States of America established
Confederates fired on Fort Sumter
First Battle of Bull Run

1862: Homestead Act
Lincoln issued Emancipation Proclamation

1863: West Virginia became 35th state
Battle of Gettysburg; Lincoln's Gettysburg Address

1864: Nevada became 36th state
Sherman marched to the sea

1865: Lee surrendered to Grant
Lincoln assassinated by Booth; Andrew Johnson became President
13th Amendment abolished slavery

1866: Ku Klux Klan formed secretly

1867: Nebraska became 37th state
Seward bought Alaska for $7.2 million

1868: Johnson impeachment fails;
Grant elected President
14th Amendment granted Negroes citizenship

1869: Knights of Labor formed
Transcontinental railroad completed

1860

1860: Bellevue Hospital Medical College was founded.

1860: First children's clinic in the U.S. was opened at New York Medical College. The originator was Abraham Jacobi (1830-1919), founder of pediatrics in the United States and editor of the *American Journal of Obstetrics*.

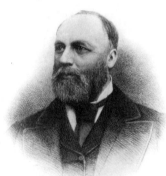

Dr. William A. Hammond

1861: The United States Sanitary Commission was created, to remedy the disorganized and inefficient state of the Union Army Medical Corps. Dr. William A. Hammond was appointed Surgeon-General.

1861: Dorothea Dix was appointed Superintendent of Nurses for the Union Army.

1862: The Confederacy gave women nurses official status.

1863: The National Academy of Sciences was founded.

1863: Two years after the Civil War began, ambulances and hospitals for wounded soldiers were put into service. Neither army had foreseen the alarming number of casualties. The Confederate Medical Corps, developed by Dr. Samuel Preston Moore, suffered from inefficient transporation systems. Until the Battle of Gettysburg, the Union Medical Corps was unable to remove its wounded from the battlefield at the end of each day's fighting.

1864: Dr. Mary Edwards Walker was commissioned Assistant Surgeon in the U.S. Army, the first woman to receive such a commission. Walker (1832-1919), was later awarded a medal for her services as a wartime surgeon.

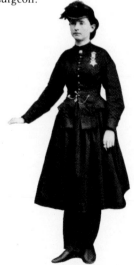

Lt. Mary Walker

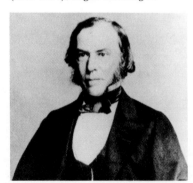

Surgeons of the 164th New York Infantry

1864: The founder of endocrinology, Charles Edouard Brown-Sequard (1817-1894), began teaching at

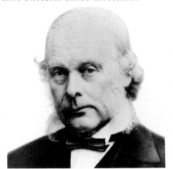

Dr. Charles Edouard Brown-Sequard

Harvard. A French-American physiologist, and an originator of organotherapy, Brown-Sequard practiced medicine in New York City from 1873 to 1878, then returned to France. He did his most important work on internal secretions (later to be called hormones), and demonstrated that these secretions could be used in treatment.

1865: Antisepsis was proved effective by English surgeon Joseph Lister (1827-1912). Lister's methods, using carbolic acid as the antiseptic agent, founded modern antiseptic surgery. His work proved Pasteur's theory that bacteria cause infection.

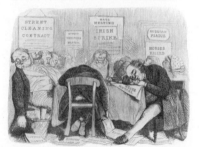

Dr. Joseph Lister

1866: The pharmaceutical firm of Parke, Davis and Company was founded by Herbey Parke and George Davis in Detroit.

1866: The Metropolitan Health Board was created in New York City. Fear of another imminent epidemic of cholera led to its establishment.

Cartoon of the New York Board of Health

60

1870: 39,818,000 inhabitants; 25.7% urban, 74.3% rural

15th Amendment gave Negroes the vote

1871: Great Chicago fire

1872: Grant reelected President

Amnesty Act restored civil rights to Southerners

1873: Record 459,803 immigrants entered U.S.

1873-78: Banks failed; Depression

1875: Sioux War began

Civil Rights Act; equal rights to Negroes

1876: Custer killed at Little Big Horn

Colorado became 38th state

Alexander Graham Bell patented the telephone

1876-77: Sioux War ended

1877: Rutherford Hayes declared President by special electoral commission

1878: Edison invented incandescent bulb

1879: National Guard Association formed

1870   **1879**

1867: Canadian Medical Association was established.

1867: One of the first out-patient departments in the U.S. was established at Bellevue Hospital, New York City. It was known as the "Bureau of Medical and Surgical Relief for the Out-door Poor."

1868: Presbyterian Hospital in New York City was founded by James Lenox, philanthropist and bibliophile.

1868: A pharmacy course initiated at the University of Michigan changed education in pharmacy. Apprenticeship as a requirement was abandoned, while innovations included laboratory work, a curriculum in basic sciences, and full-time attendance by students.

1869: University of Michigan established a temporary 20-bed hospital in a remodeled residence for clinical instruction of medical students. This makeshift teaching hospital was the first to be established under the control of a university medical school. It functioned until 1877, when a proper hospital took its place.

1869: Massachusetts became the second state to form a state board of health. The first had been created in Louisiana in 1855.

1869: The *American Journal of Obstetrics* was founded.

1870: U.S. Public Health Service was established. It became the principal federal health agency, gradually merging its functions with those of the Marine Hospital Service established a century earlier.

1872: The American Public Health Association was founded.

1872: Hay fever was first described by Morrill Wyman of Cambridge, Massachusetts.

1873: The first modern American school of nursing, patterned on the plan suggested by Florence Nightingale (1820-1910), of England, was established at Bellevue Hospital, New York City. Similar schools, designed primarily to give nurses professional training rather than to provide nursing service for the hospital, were established the same year in Boston and New Haven.

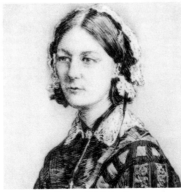

Florence Nightingale

1874: University of Pennsylvania established the first full-fledged university hospital in the U.S.

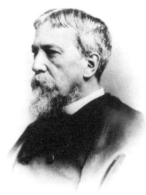

Dr. S. Weir Mitchell

1875: The "rest cure" was introduced by S. Weir Mitchell (1829-1914).

1875: Lydia Pinkham of Lynn, Massachusetts, began to make and sell her Vegetable Compound. This famous patent medicine was advertised as a "positive cure for all those painful complaints and weaknesses so common to our best female population."

1876: Colonel Eli Lilly began his pharmaceutical manufacturing business in Indianapolis.

1877: The U.S. Pharmacopoeia Revision Committee was modified at the convention of the American Pharmaceutical Association.

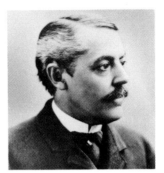

Colonel Eli Lilly

1878: Dr. J. Marion Sims performed the first gall bladder operation.

1879: Mary E.P. Mahoney, the first black nurse in the U.S., graduated from the nursing school at the New England Hospital for Women and Children, Boston.

1879: Listerine Antiseptic was formulated by Jordan Wheat Lambert of St. Louis. Named in honor of Joseph Lister, the antiseptic became available in every drug, food, and variety store in the country after the Lambert Company was formed in 1884.

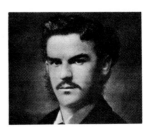

Jordan Lambert

61

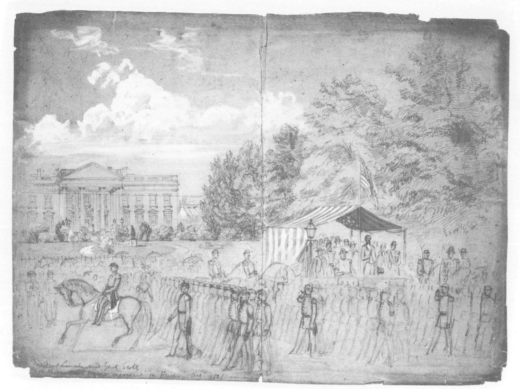

Left: A Union Regiment Reviewed by President Lincoln. Print, 1861. [L.C.] As North and South divided, so did America's medical community. After John Brown's raid in 1859, almost 200 Southern medical students quit Philadelphia colleges for Richmond's Medical College of Virginia. *Below:* The Harewood Hospital, Washington. Lithograph, 19th century. [N.L.M.] The Union and Confederacy quickly erected or converted buildings for medical service.

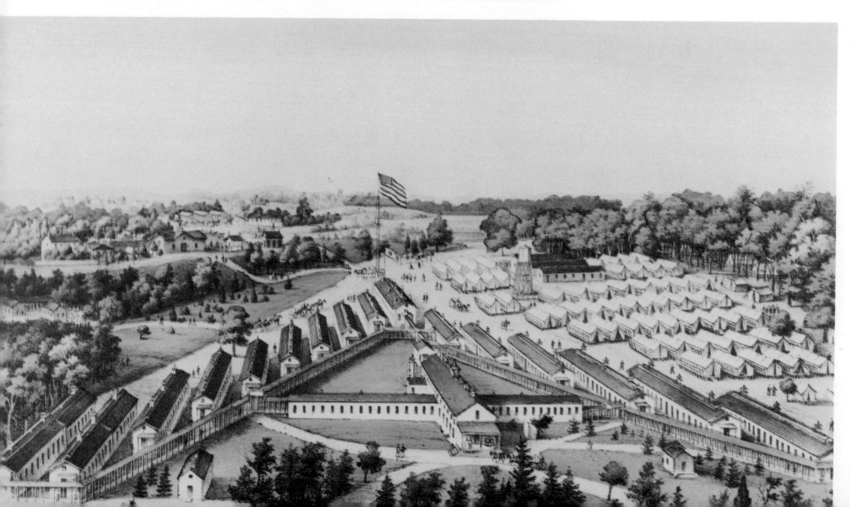

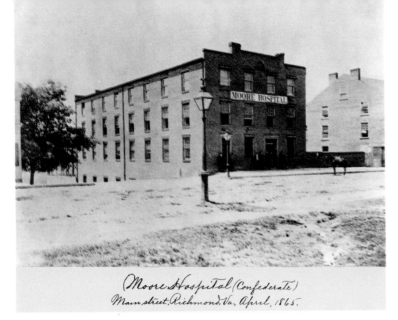

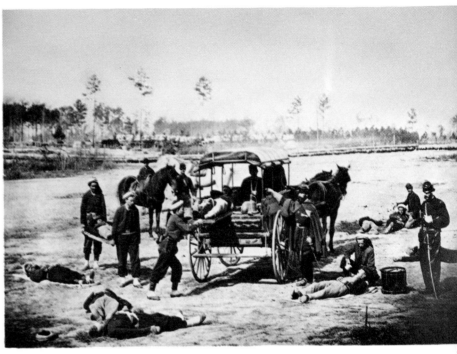

Above: Moore Hospital (Confederate). Daguerreotype, 19th century. [L.C.] This Richmond hospital was tiny in comparison to the city's Chimborazo Hospital, which was completed in 1861. *Right:* Ambulance Drill. Daguerreotype, 1864. [L.C.] Medical corpsmen of the Union Army. *Below:* Union Surgeons of Seminary Hospital, Georgetown, D.C. Daguerreotype, 19th century. [L.C.]

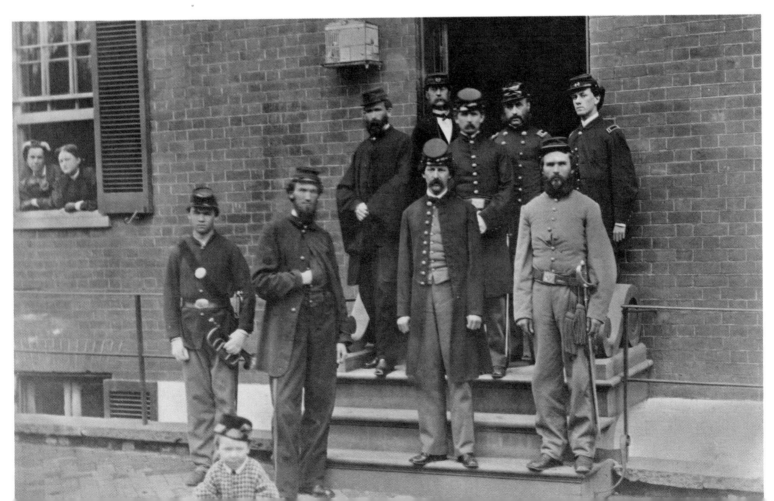

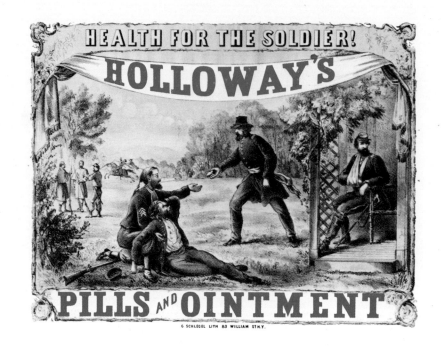

GREAT EXCITEMENT
IN
South Carolina!

Was being caused before the war by the wonderful cures of Bronchitis, Asthma, Sore Throat, Consumption, &c., &c., effected by Wishart's Pine Tree Tar Cordial, in and around Charleston.

BEAUREGARD

himself might as well be

A PRISONER!

as to be confined with a distressing Cough or Sore Throat and not be able to obtain Wishart's Pine Tree Tar Cordial, which is known to cure all Complaints of the Throat, Consumption, &c.

Depot, No. 10 North Second Street.

Above: Wishart's Pine Tree Tar Cordial. Advertising broadside. Print, 1863. [L.C.]
Right: Holloway's Pills and Ointment. Advertising broadside. Print, 1863. [L.C.] Patent medicine purveyors adapted readily to wartime.

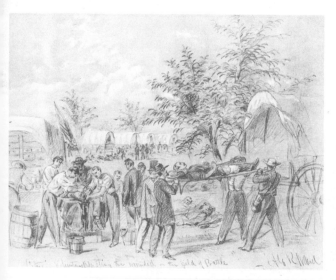

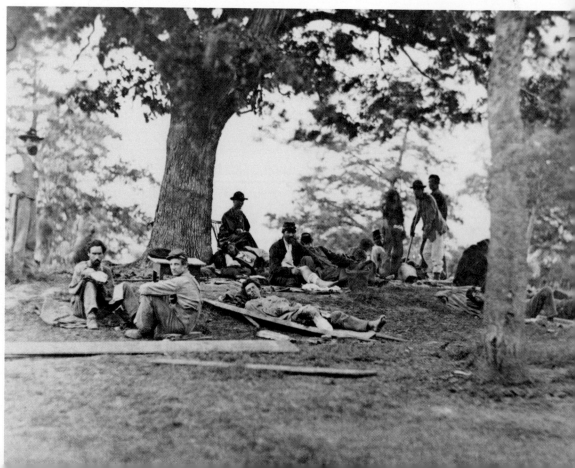

Above: Carrying in the Wounded at Bull Run. Drawing, 1861. [N.L.M.] From the onset of the Civil War, *Harper's Weekly* provided graphic coverage of all its aspects.
Right: Wounded Soldiers After the Battle of Chancellorsville. Daguerreotype, 1863. [N.A.]

64

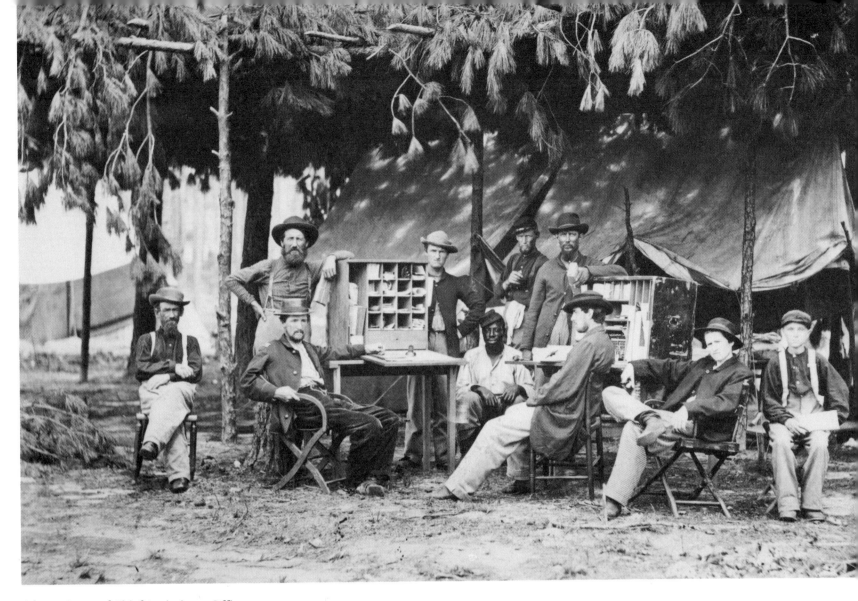

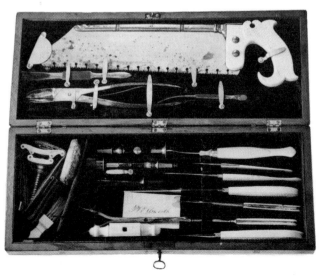

Above: Camp of Chief Ambulance Officer, 9th Army Corps. Daguerreotype, August, 1864. [L.C.] This group portrait was made at a field hospital near Petersburg, Virginia.
Right: Cased Surgical Kit. Mixed materials, 1860. [H.M.S.] This was carried by Pinchney Webster Ellsworth, M.D.

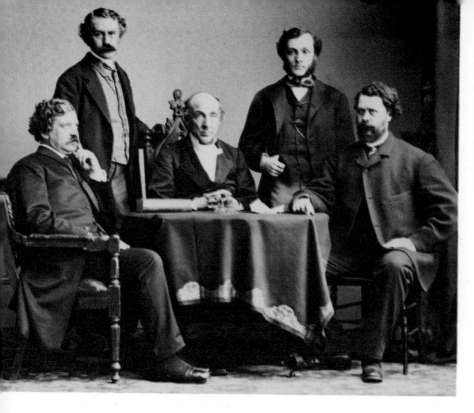

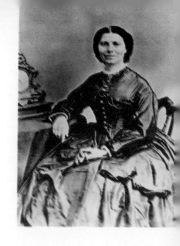

Left: The United States Sanitary Commission. Daguerreotype, 1861. [L.C.]
Right: Clara Barton. Daguerreotype by Matthew Brady, 1866. [N.A.] Clara Barton founded the American Red Cross in 1881, and served as a nurse in the Civil War.
Below: Dorothea Dix. Daguerreotype, c. 1850. [L.C.]

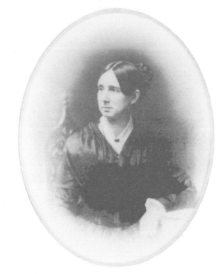

Below right: Civil War Nurses. Daguerreotype, c. 1865. [M.17.]
Below Left: Field Outfit of the Sanitary Commission. Daguerreotype, c. 1860s. [L.C]

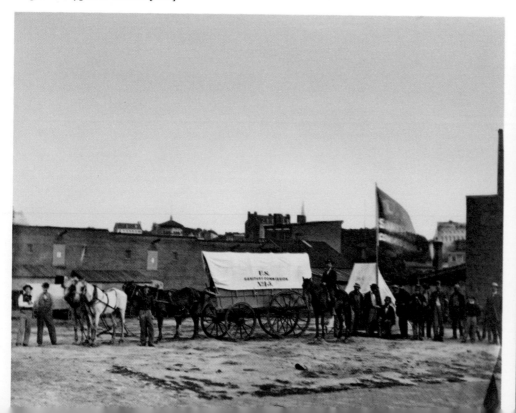

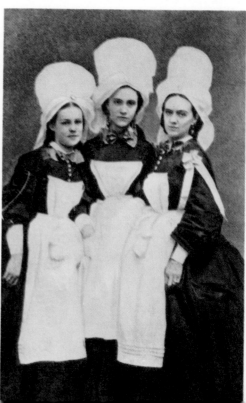

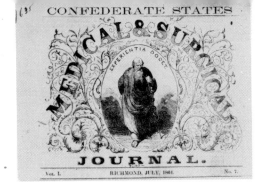

Left: Masthead of the *Confederate States Medical and Surgical Journal.* Print, 1864. [N.Y.P.L./P.C.] Published in Richmond, Virginia.

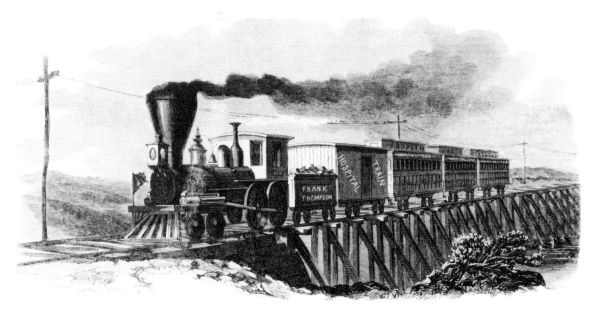

Above: Hospital Train from Chattanooga to Nashville. Engraving, c. 1864. [C.H.M.] As the war progressed, so did the efficiency of the Medical Corps of the Union Army. This particular train was under the care of Dr. Myers. *Right:* Interior of a Hospital Car. Engraving, c. 1864. [C.H.M.] Following a surgeon's advice, the beds were suspended from India rubber bands attached to the car's framework. As the beds yielded to the train's motion, the wounded were less jostled.

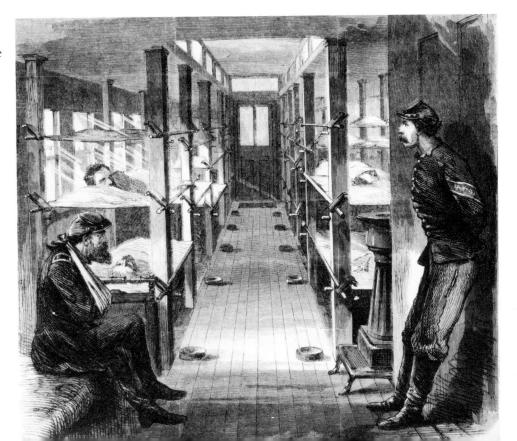

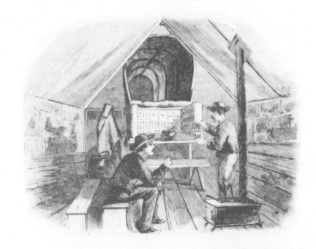

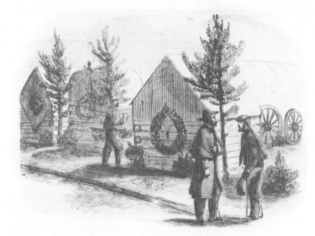

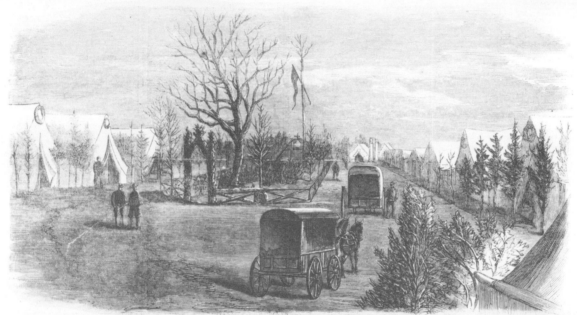

Views of a U.S. Army Field Hospital.
Engravings. 1865. [C.H.M.] *Harper's Weekly*
hired Mr. A. McCullum, an English artist, to
make these sketches of the hospital of the First
Division of the 9th Corps. *Above left:* Interior
of a Hospital Supply Tent and Wagon. *Above
right:* Exterior View of Hospital Tent. *Middle:*
A General View of the Hospital. *Right:*
Operating Room. *Far right:* Interior of a
Hospital Ward.

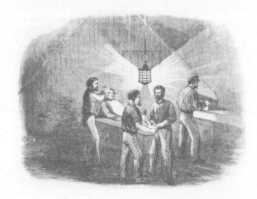

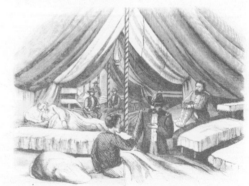

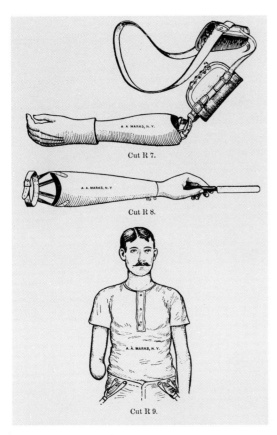

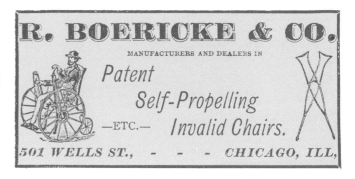

Left: Artificial Arm. Page from a stock book, late 19th century.[M.18.]. *Right:* Advertisement, Self-Propelling Invalid Chairs. Print, c. 1870s. [N.M.H.T.] *Below:* Three Feeding Devices. *Top:* Porcelain [M.J.] *Bottom two:* Pewter, 19th century. [P.C.]

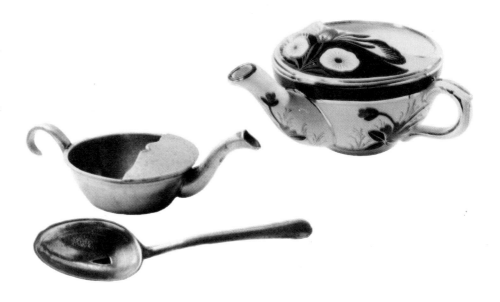

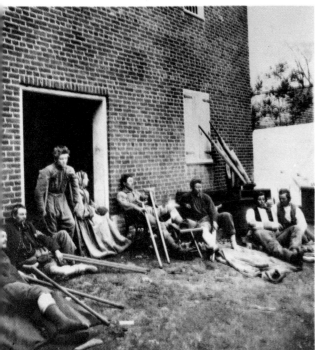

Left: Union Soldiers Wounded at Fredericksburg Following Battle of May 3, 1863. Photograph by Matthew Brady. [M.18.] Although the Civil War records are not precise, the North reported 359,528 killed and 246,712 wounded, and the South 258,000 killed and 200,000 wounded. *Below:* A View of a Hospital Ward. Daguerreotype by Matthew Brady, 1866. [N.A.]

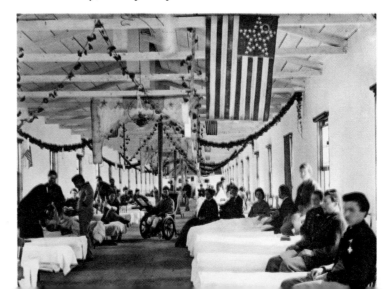

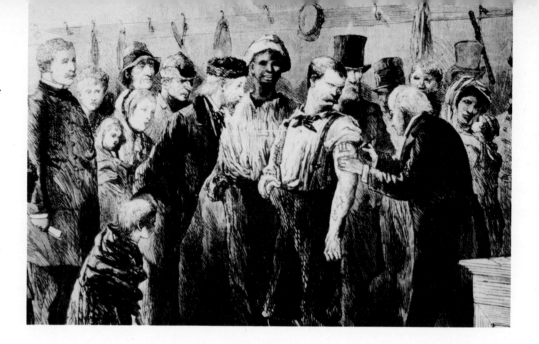

Right: Vaccinating the Poor, Print, c. 1872. [N.L.M] This illustration appeared in *Harper's Weekly.*

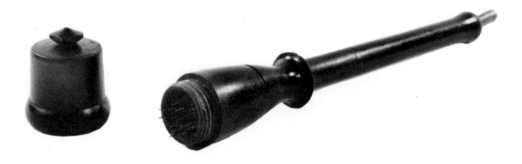

Above center: Scarifier. Ebony, 19th century. [H.M.M.] This device was used for vaccinating. *Left:* Vaccination. Print, 1872. [C.H.M.] Dr. Chambon vaccinating patients in his parlor with virus taken directly from the animal. *Harper's Weekly* captioned this illustration, ''The Smallpox Excitement.''

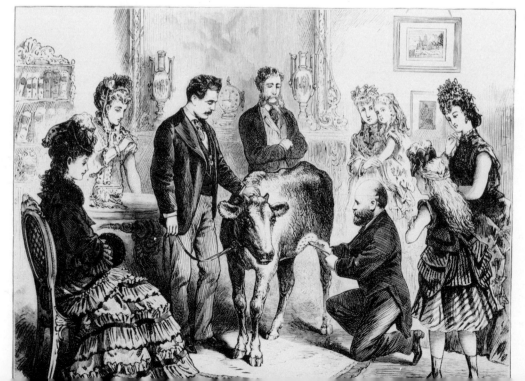

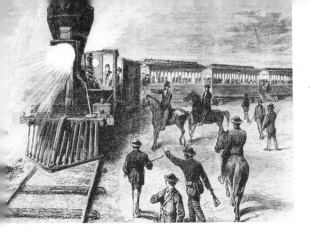

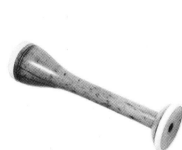

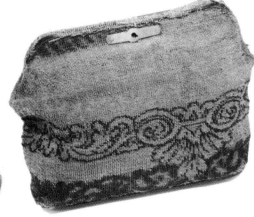

Left: Health Officers Quarantining a Train. Print, 1873. [C.H.M.] This event occurred near Dallas, Texas during the yellow fever outbreak in 1873. *Below:* Stethoscope. Wood, c. 1860. [H.M.M.] *Right:* Medical Bag. Carpet covered, 19th century. [H.M.M.]

Below: The Sick Women in Bellevue Hospital, New York, Overrun by Rats. Print, 1860. [N.L.M.] The atmosphere in many 19th century city hospitals was distinctly unappealing. In 1872 a visitor to Bellevue described the state of the beds and patients as ''unspeakable. The one nurse slept in the bathroom and the tub was filled with filthy rubbish.''

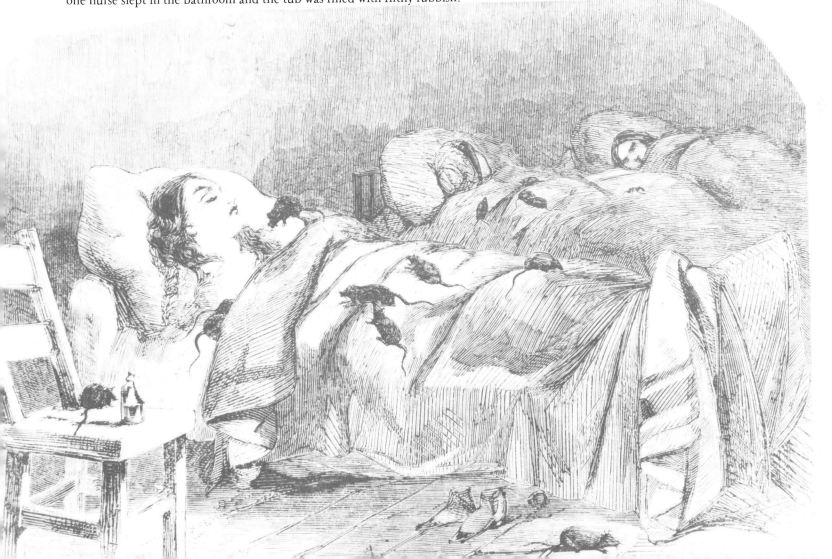

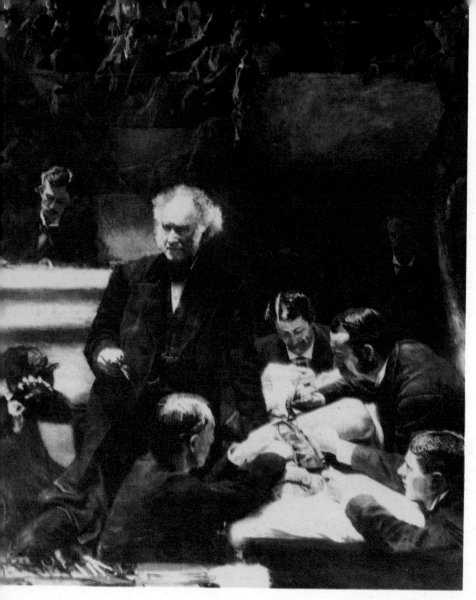

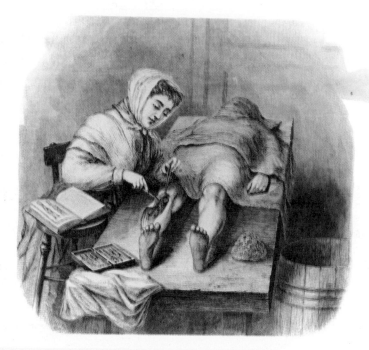

Left: The Gross Clinic. Painting by Thomas Eakins, 1875. [M.19.] At this time operations by such brilliant surgeons and teachers as Dr. Samuel Gross of Philadelphia were performed with unwashed hands, instruments that had not been disinfected, and dirty sponges and bandages. The resulting mortality rate due to sepsis was very high.

Above right: Dissection by a Woman Medical Student. Engraving, 1870. [N.L.M.] *Right:* Anatomy Lesson. Print, wood, 1870. [N.Y.P.L./P.C.] Medical education included more and more women. On the right an instructor is seen teaching anatomy to a class at New York Medical College for Women, founded in 1870, while the student above is dissecting the leg of a cadaver.

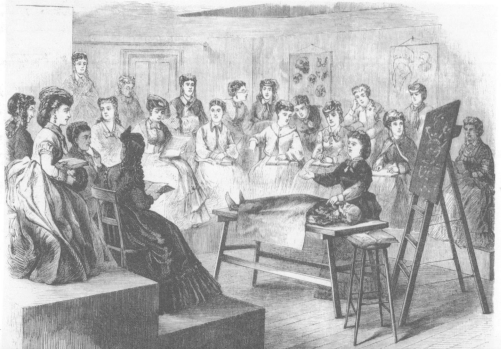

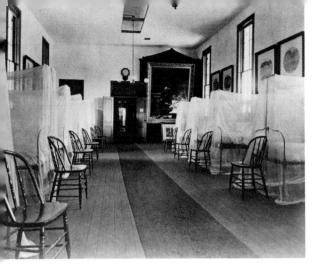 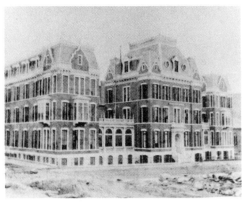 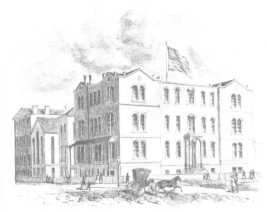

Above left: First Aid Hospital Exhibit at 1876 Centennial Exposition, Philadelphia. Photograph. [L.C.] The great Eakins' painting, ''The Gross Clinic,'' is seen in the background. *Above center:* Mt. Sinai Hospital. Photograph, late 19th century. [M.4.] *Above right:* The Nursery and Child's Hospital. Print, late 19th century. [C.H.M.] *Below:* The Presbyterian Hospital. Photograph, 1872. [M.20.] New York City's hospitals were becoming specialized, as these views indicate. The building's exteriors also reveal the range of Victorian architectural style then fashionable.

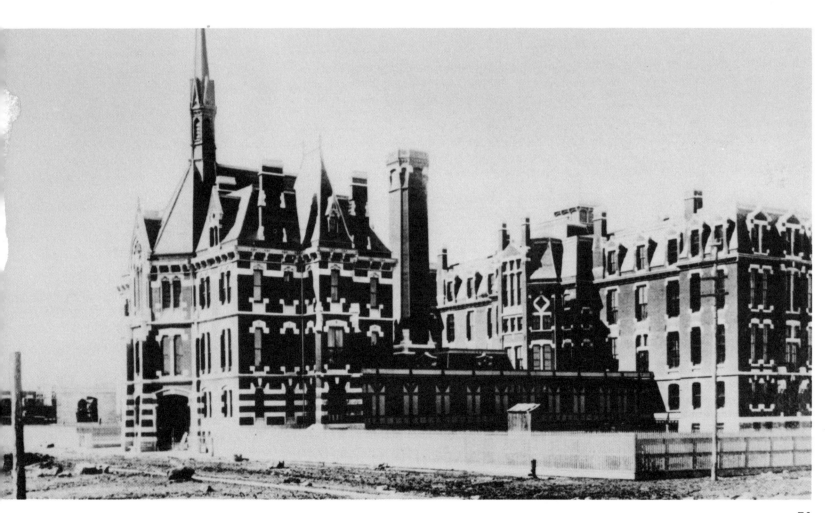

Below: General George Custer. Engraving by Frederick Remington after a daguerreotype by Matthew Brady, c. 1875. [P.C.] Custer and over 200 members of his 7th Cavalry were killed in the Battle of Little Big Horn on June 25, 1876 by the Sioux and Cheyenne. *Center:* Medicine Bag, Medicine Man's Stick with Arrow. Mixed materials, 19th century. [P.C.P.S.] The medicine bag, made of an animal scrotum, contained medicinal herbs and was worn by a Cheyenne brave around his neck.

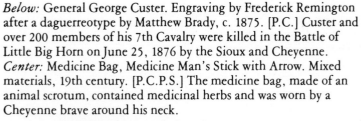

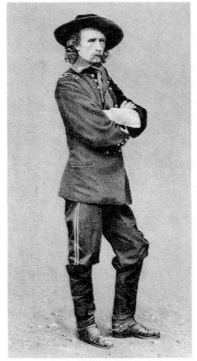

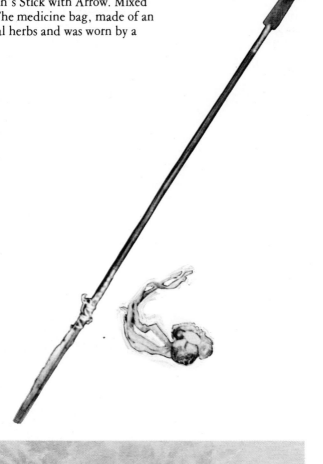

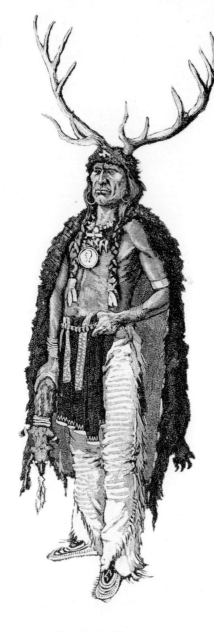

Above: Medicine Elk. Engraving after Frederick Remington, c. 1875. [P.C.] Medicine Elk was a shaman of the Oglala Sioux. *Left:* Improvised Stretcher. Engraving, 1876. [N.L.M.] Wounded in the Indian Wars were frequently transported to hospitals by horse stretchers.

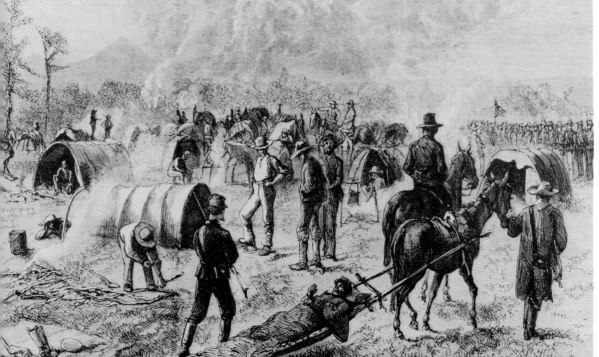

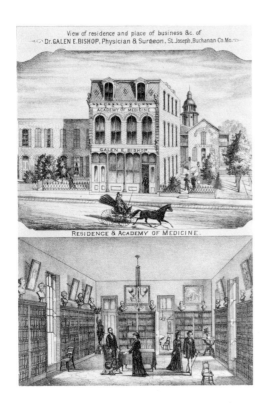

Left: Residence and Academy of Medicine. Print, 1879. [L.C.] Dr. Galen E. Bishop was a physician of St. Joseph, Mo., who according to *The Atlas of Andrew Co., Mo.,* "founded an institution . . . that is an honor to the city and the State." It is not known if the Academy was in fact one of the unaccredited license mills then in existence. *Below right:* The Country Doctor. Engraving after a drawing by A.R. Waud, 1869. [L.C.]

Below: Pioneer Birth Scene. Engraving 1887. [N.L.M.] An American pioneer woman in labor sits on her husband's lap grasping the hands of two midwives, who sit across from her, bracing and helping her. In effect, the husband acts as a "birth stool."

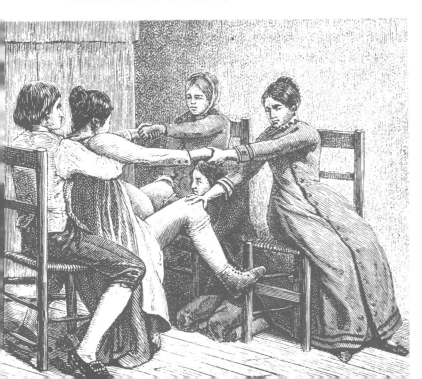

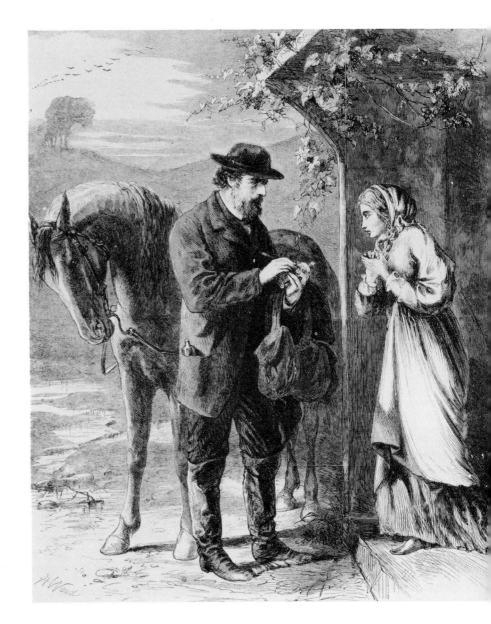

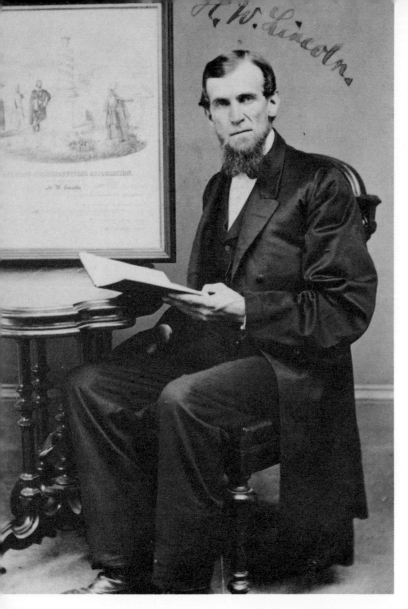

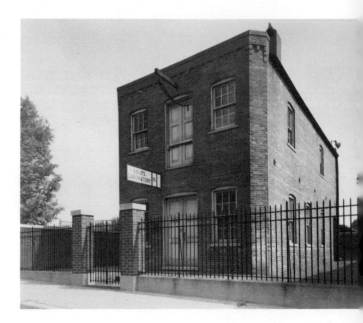

Left: Dr. Henry W. Lincoln. Daguerreotype, c. 1865. [A.P.A.] Dr. Lincoln, of Boston, was president of the American Pharmaceutical Association from 1865 to 1866. The Association's certificate is on the wall behind him. *Below:* Lilly's Laboratory. [E.L.] An exact replica of the original laboratory, erected in 1934 in Indianapolis.

Below: A.Ph.A. Convention. Daguerreotype. [A.P.A.] This national convention was held in Cleveland, Ohio, in 1872.

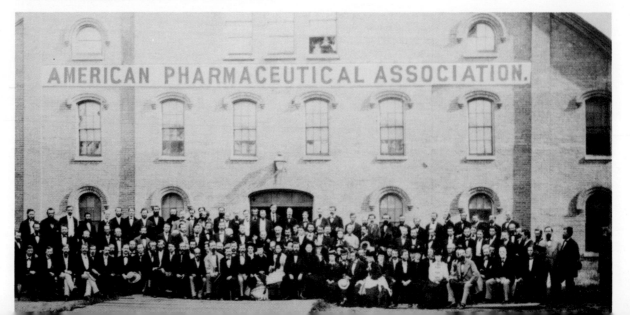

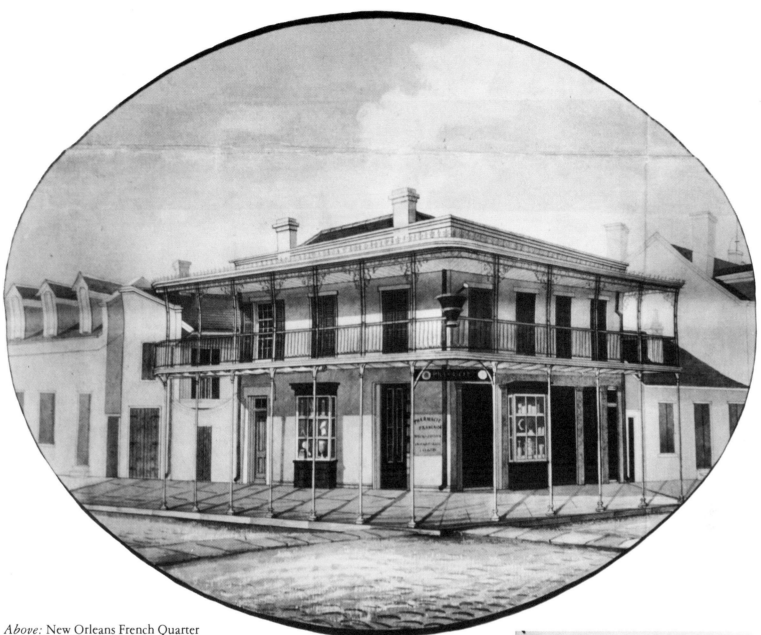

Above: New Orleans French Quarter Pharmacy. Watercolor, mid 19th century. [P.C.] The pharmacist and his family probably lived on the second floor. *Right:* C.A. Marsh's Drugstore. Photograph, 1865. [M.C.N.Y.] A New York City drugstore at 125th Street and Third Avenue. *Far right:* Quackinbush and Son. Daguerreotype, 19th Century. [P.C.] This New York City store proudly proclaimed, "Founded February 22, 1817."

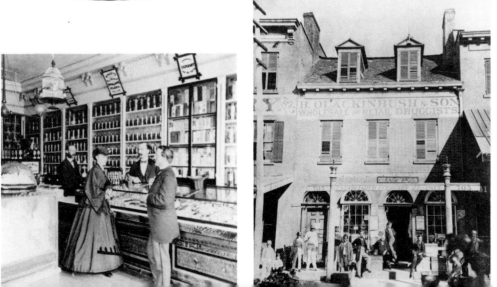

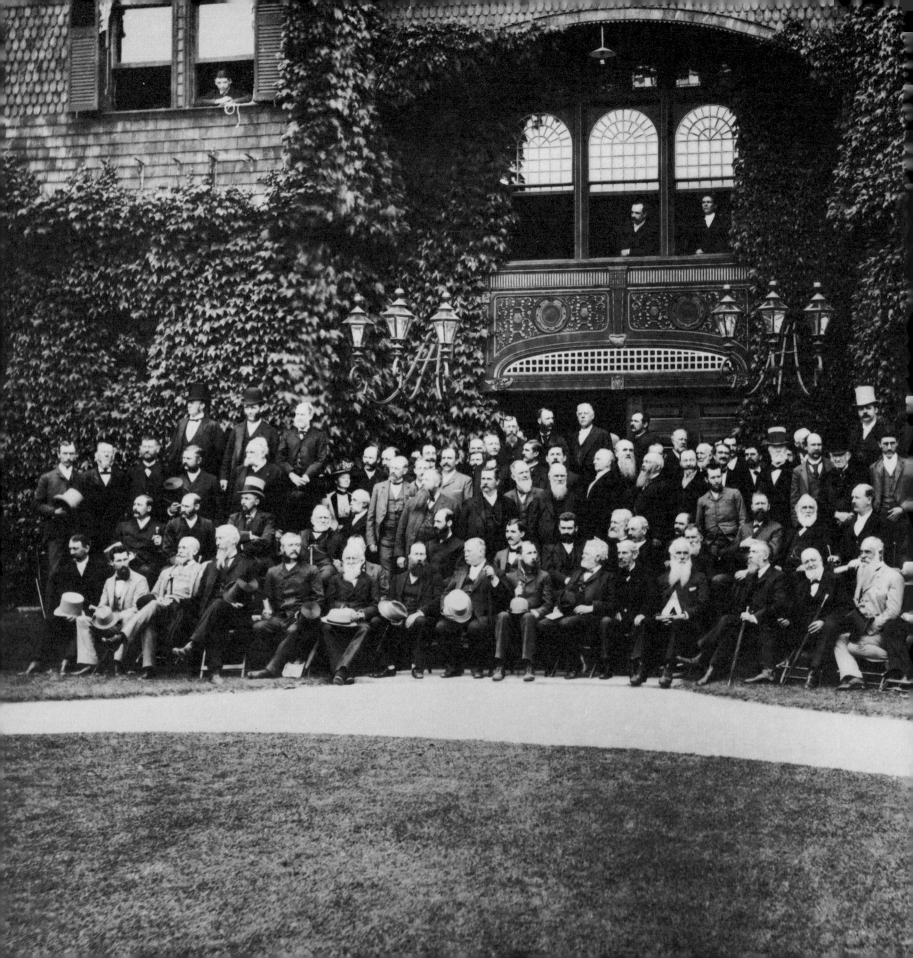

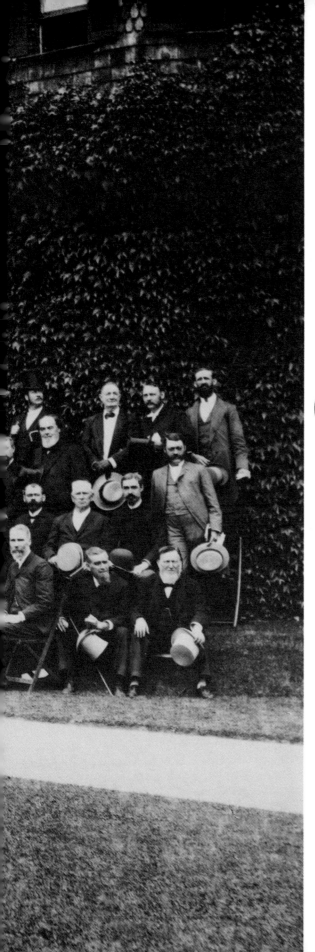

CHAPTER FIVE

1880-1899

On July 15, 1884, Mark Twain wrote his friend, William Dean Howells, about his arduous experience with the dentist, Dr. John M. Riggs, of Hartford, Connecticut, a pioneer in the burgeoning field of periodontal pathology. "I have been in the dental chair ten days, a couple of hours a day. The dentist is a bright man, & gouges & digs & saws & rasps & Hammers, & keeps up a steady stream of entertaining talk, all the time, like his professional ancestor the barber." Prior to the 1840s, dentistry was practiced in the main by barbers, jewelers, blacksmiths and itinerant quacks. However, by 1900, American dentistry had achieved world-renowned and professional status.

The 19th century witnessed the growth of yet another previously ignored field, public health. Massive European immigration meant overcrowded cities and recurrent epidemics. The need for effective public health organizations became acute.

In 1886 the first such administration was created, followed by state and municipal health departments throughout the country which contributed greatly to the prevention and control of communicable diseases and to improved sanitary conditions and child hygiene. Public health ceased to be an individual responsibility and became a government obligation.

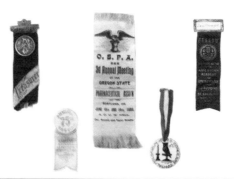

Left: American Medical Association Convention. Photograph, 1889. [A.M.A.] By the summer of 1889, when its national convention was held in Newport, Rhode Island, the A.M.A. had grown to a membership of 4,346 (out of an estimated 80,000 physicians in the country). *Above:* Medical Societies' Convention Badges. Mixed materials, late 19th and early 20th centuries. [P.C.P.S.]

1880: Census showed 50,155,000 inhabitants
James A. Garfield elected President

1881: Garfield assassinated; Chester Arthur
became President
American Red Cross organized

1881-90: 5,246,613 immigrants entered U.S.

1882: U.S. subscribed to Geneva Convention

1883: Pendleton Act created Civil Service
Commission

1884: Grover Cleveland elected President
U.S. Bureau of Labor created

1884-88: Equal Rights Party formed by
Suffragettes

1885: Chicago's Home Insurance Building dubbed
a "skyscraper"

1886: American Federation of Labor formed
Statue of Liberty dedicated

1887: First federal regulatory agency,
Interstate Commerce Commission

1888: Benjamin Harrison elected President
George Eastman marketed first box camera

1889: North Dakota, South Dakota,
Montana, Washington became 39,
40th, 41st, 42nd states

1880

1881: Entrance examinations as a requirement for admission to medical school were first introduced at the University of Pennsylvania.

1881: Alexander Graham Bell devised an electrical detector to locate the assassin's bullet in the body of the dying President, James Garfield. This was among the first of many contributions made by electricity to medicine.

1881: American Red Cross was organized by Clara Barton (1821-1912). In the Civil War, Barton, a former teacher and government clerk, had nursed in army camps and at the scene of fighting, where she was called "the Angel of the Battlefield." President Lincoln appointed her to search for missing prisoners, and her records identified thousands of Union dead at Andersonville. She headed the American Red Cross until 1904, emphasizing relief work in catastrophes as well as wars.

1882: The bacillus causing tuberculosis was discovered by Robert Koch (1843-1910), of Germany. It became clear that tuberculosis, a major cause of death in the 19th century, spread through close personal contact. In 1884 the first modern tuberculosis sanatorium was founded at Saranac Lake in the Adirondacks by Edward Trudeau (1848-1915), a physician who himself suffered from the illness. Open-air treatment was given. In 1894 the first laboratory for the study of tuberculosis was organized there.

1884: Dr. W.E. Upjohn, a young physician from Michigan, developed the "friable" pill which would readily dissolve. Two years later, with his brother Dr. Henry Upjohn, he founded The Upjohn Pill and Granule Company in Kalamazoo.

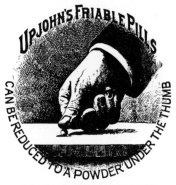

Advertisement, Upjohn's Friable Pills

1885: The first visiting nurse service began work in Buffalo, New York.

1885: A clergyman founded what is now the Norwich-Eaton Pharmaceutical Company. The Reverend Lafayette F. Moore, minister of several churches in upstate New York, settled in Norwich and began to manufacture pills for physicians in the Chenango river valley.

1886: The three Johnson brothers formed a partnership and began to manufacture plasters. In 1887 Johnson & Johnson incorporated, and started making dressings and antiseptic ligatures.

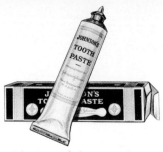

Advertisement, Johnson's Tooth Paste

1886: Appendicitis (formerly known as typhlitis) was identified and named. Reginald H. Fitz (1843-1913), of Boston first clearly described the signs and symptoms by which a diagnosis could be made. After this, surgeons began to diagnose appendicitis with increasing accuracy and appendectomy became the most common abdominal operation.

1887: John Ripley Myers and William McLaren Bristol founded the Bristol-Myers company in Clinton, New York. Originally named the Clinton Pharmaceutical Company, the firm incorporated as Bristol-Myers in 1900. Sal Hepatica, initially called Clinton Salts, was an early product.

1887: An American branch of the pharmaceutical firm of E. Merck of Darmstadt, Germany, was established. In 1891, Merck & Co. was incorporated in New York.

1888: W.B. Saunders Company, a leading medical publisher, was founded in Philadelphia.

1889: The second great epidemic of influenza struck the United States. The first epidemic occurred a century earlier.

1889: Johns Hopkins Hospital was completed. The training school for female nurses opened five months after the hospital.

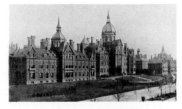

Johns Hopkins Hospital

1889: Sterile surgical gloves as a means to asepsis were introduced. At Johns Hopkins they were introduced by William Stewart Halsted (1852-1922), first professor of surgery—because his fiancee, the head operating nurse, had hands sensitive to bichloride of mercury. Not until 1894 did the treatise *Aseptic Surgical Technique* suggest that all members of surgical teams wear gloves.

1889: Mayo Clinic opened in Rochester, Minnesota, founded by William Worrall Mayo, whose two sons, Charles Horace Mayo (1865-1939), and William James Mayo (1861-1939), gained it an international reputation.

1890: U.S. Public Health Service began the inspection of immigrants.

1890: 62,947,714 inhabitants; 35.1% urban, 64.9% rural
Sherman Antitrust Act passed
Battle of Wounded Knee, South Dakota
Ellis Island opened December 31st
1891: Superintendent of Immigration established
1891-1900: 3,687,564 immigrants came to U.S.
1892: People's Party (Populists), national party
Grover Cleveland elected President
Homestead strike
1893: Ford built his first automobile
1894: Bureau of Immigration established
Labor Day declared legal holiday
Republic of Hawaii recognized by U.S.
1895: Gillette invented safety razor blade
1896: Utah became 45th state
William McKinley elected 25th President
"Separate but equal" doctrine approved by Court
1898: U.S.S. Maine blown up in Havana
Congress declared war on Spain
Battles of El Caney and San Juan Hill
Spain ceded Puerto Rico, Phillippines, Guam to U.S.
1899: U.S. declared Open Door Policy
1899-1902: Boer War

890   1899

1892: The one volume *Principles and Practice of Medicine,* one of the most prestigious textbooks of modern times, was written by Sir William Osler (1849-1919). Osler, Canadian-born physician and renowned medical historian, was the most brilliant and influential teacher of his day. He was professor at McGill (1875-1884), at the University of Pennsylvania (1884-1889), and at Johns Hopkins (1889-1904).

1892: *A Manual of Bacteriology* by George M. Sternberg was published. The systematic studies of infectious diseases by Sternberg (1838-1915), who became Surgeon-General of the Army in 1893, attracted world-wide attention. Dr. Sternberg organized successful research projects, including Walter Reed's study of yellow fever. He has been called the father of American bacteriology.

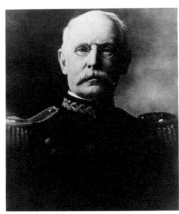

Dr. George M. Sternberg

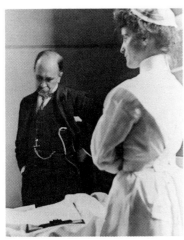

Dr. William Osler Making Ward Rounds

1893: Johns Hopkins medical school was opened. The first class included 14 men and 3 women students. In their third year, students entered the hospital to work and learn in the dispensary and wards. Close contact with patients was an educational innovation introduced by William Osler, and a great contrast to other respected schools—where a student might receive a prize in obstetrics without ever having seen a woman in labor.

1893: The first American chair in the new discipline of pharmacology was created at Johns Hopkins. The first professor was John Jacob Abel (1857-1938), who taught pharmacology until 1932, then became director of the laboratory for endocrine research.

1893: The first proof that disease could be transmitted by insects was published by Theobald Smith (1859-1934). After working with Daniel E. Salmon on hog cholera, at the Department of Agriculture's Bureau of Animal Industry, Smith proved that Texas cattle fever was caused by microorganisms carried by ticks. The discovery of insect-borne disease, one of the most important American contributions to medical knowledge, would prove to have practical applications in the control of human illnesses.

1893: Lillian Wald (1867-1940) founded the Henry Street Settlement Visiting Nurse Service. The Visiting Nurse Service, still in existence, provided home care to all patients in need, regardless of ability to pay. Lillian Wald graduated in 1891 from the New York Hospital school of nursing, spent one year as a nurse in an orphanage, and another studying at the Women's Medical College of the New York Infirmary before beginning this public service.

1894: First large epidemic of poliomyelitis struck the United States.

1895: A specific antitoxin, developed in Europe, revolutionized treatment of diphtheria. The serum, produced in the U.S. by Parke, Davis and other companies, saved the lives of thousands of children.

1896: The Nurses' Associated Alumni formed. In 1911 this became the American Nurses Association.

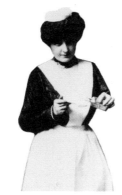

A Nurse of the Late 19th Century

1896: X-ray treatment was first used. Discovered in late 1895 by Wilhelm Roentgen (1845-1923), of Germany, radiographs had immediate medical applications.

1896: Antityphoid inoculation was introduced. Mass inoculations began in the first decade of the 20th century.

1898: Epinephrin was isolated from the adrenal glands, in a lab at Johns Hopkins. The pharmacologist John Jacob Abel (1857-1938), isolated the valuable hormone commonly known today as adrenalin.

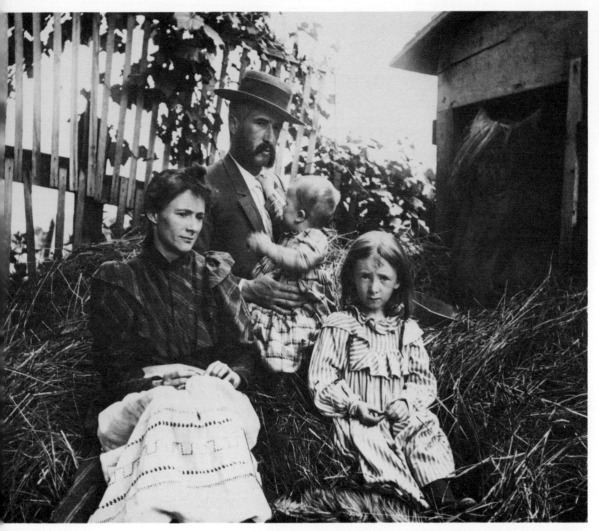

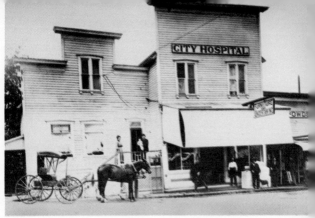

Left: Dr. Edward A. Bass with Family and Horse. Photograph, 1881. [S.H.S.W.] Dr. Bass practiced medicine around Montello, Wisconsin, between 1870 and 1900. The reverse side of this photograph bears the notation, "The horse's name is Dick."
Above: City Hospital. Photograph, 1900. [M.22.] Drs. Katherine and Henry Schleef established the first hospital in Cottage Grove, Oregon. *Below:* Physician's Bag. Mixed materials, c. 1895. [H.M.S.] The contents indicate this was the bag of a "general practitioner."

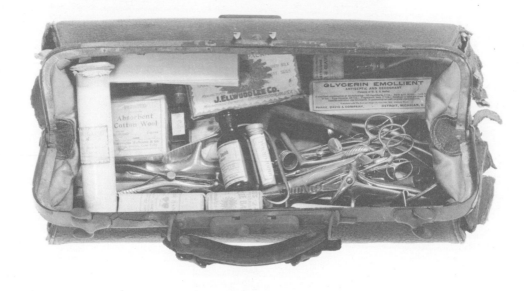

Right: A Board of Health Doctor. Engraving, 1895. [N.Y.A.M.] As epidemics occurred more frequently in the growing cities, city health efforts intensified. Here a doctor visits a patient in a New York City tenement. *Far right:* Disinfecting Corps. Engraving, 1884. [N.Y.A.M.] Board of Health officials at work in the basement of a slum lodging house during a heat wave. *Below:* A Suspected Cholera Victim. Engraving, 1890s. [N.Y.A.M.] Patient is being helped from a slum building to an awaiting ambulance.

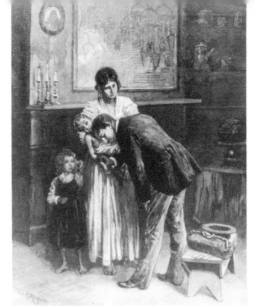

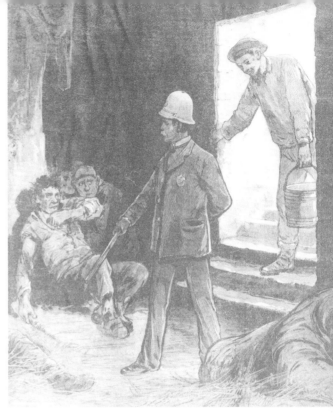

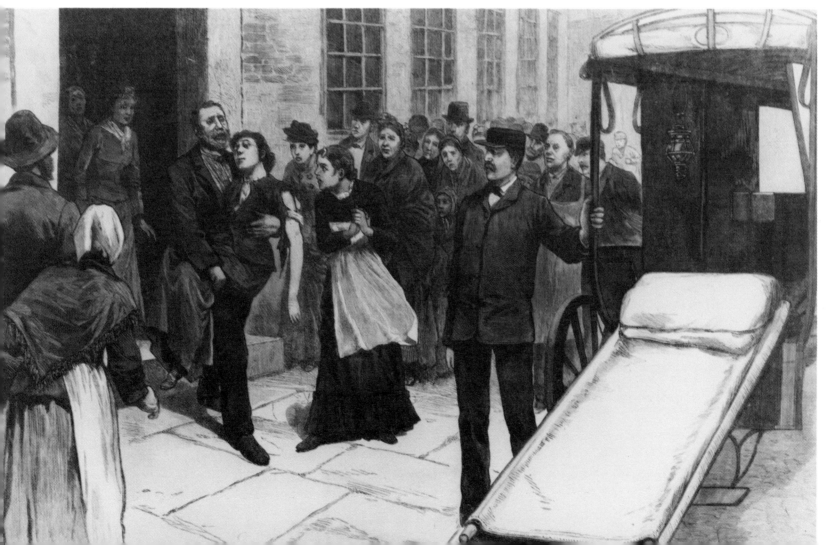

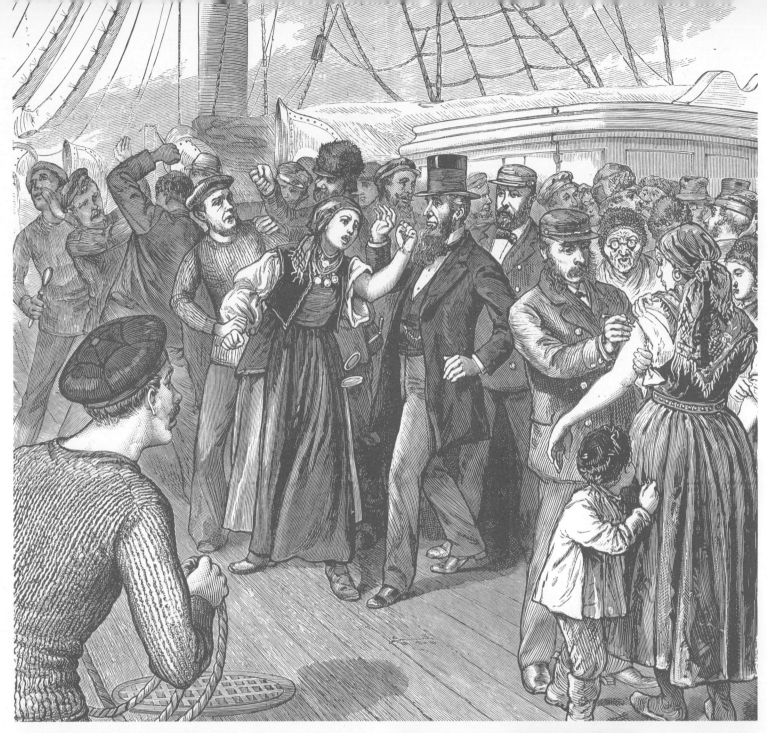

Above: Vaccinating Immigrants. Engraving, 1881. [L.C.] New York City health officers are shown on board the quarantined *Victoria*, persuading Russian and Polish immigrants to submit to vaccination.
Right: Patients Turned Over to a Receiving Hospital. Photograph, 1892. [N.Y.C.D.H.] Immigrants with contagious diseases were removed from a quarantined ship to a hospital on New York City's North Brother Island.

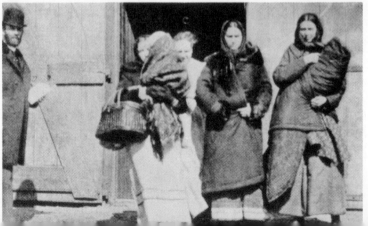

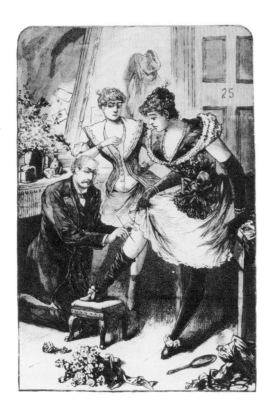

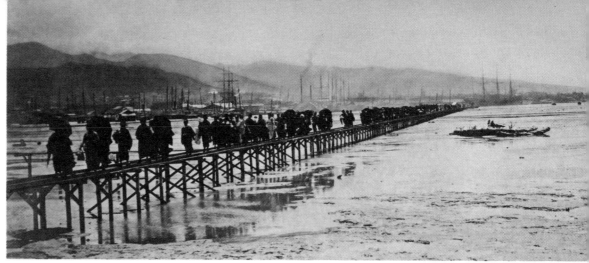

Left: Performance Stopped to Vaccinate Players. Engraving, c. 1880s. [F.L.I.] "Gala night for vaccine lymph in Boston," says the caption of this *Police Gazette* illustration. *Above:* Chinese Immigrants Leave Quarantine in San Francisco. Photograph, 1890. [N.A.] By the end of the 19th century, people from four corners of the world were crowding into American cities. *Below left:* An Incident in Montreal. Engraving, 1885. [C.H.M.] French Canadians knew, as did citizens of all North American cities, that children taken away in "the Small-Pox Van" seldom returned. *Below right:* Fighting Tuberculosis on the Roof. Photograph by Jacob A. Riis, 1890. [P.C.] From his famous photographic exposé, *How the Other Half Lives*.

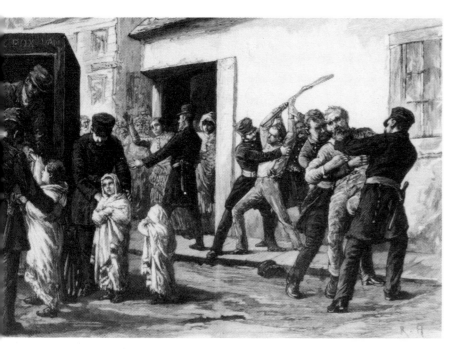

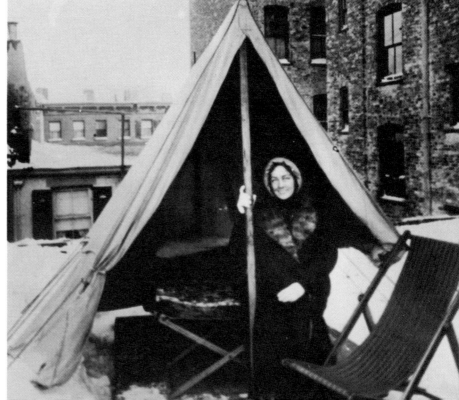

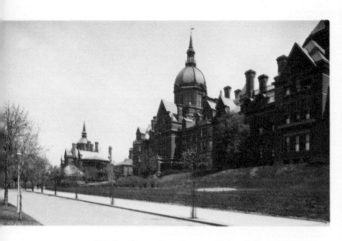

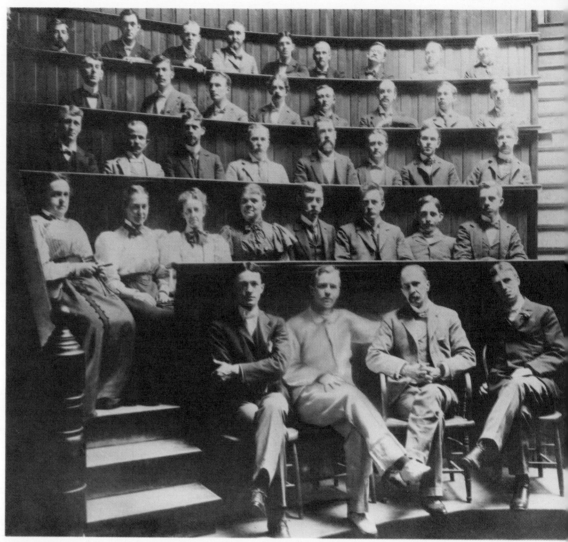

Right: Post-Graduate Class, Johns Hopkins University School of Medicine. Photograph, late 1890s. [N.L.M.] Four in this class of thirty-four students were women.
Foreground left to right: Drs. Harvey Williams Cushing; Howard A. Kelly and William Osler, two of the four founders of the School of Medicine; W.S. Thayer. *Above:* The Johns Hopkins Hospital. Photograph, 1889. [N.L.M.] *Below left:* Grave Robbers. Engraving, 1892. [F.L.I.] The *Police Gazette* caption: ''For the Dissecting Table. The body of Miss Cassell dragged from its grave in Indianapolis, Ind., by embryo doctors.''
Below right: Operation for Radical Mastectomy, Yale-New Haven Hospital, New Haven, Conn. Photograph, 1894. [N.L.M.]

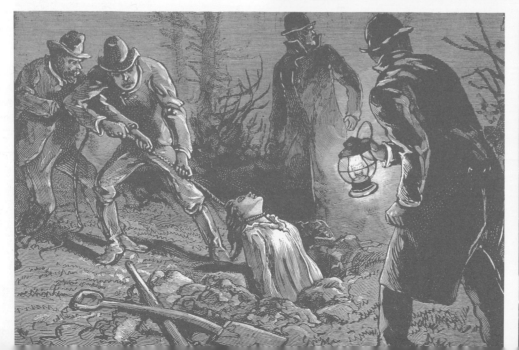

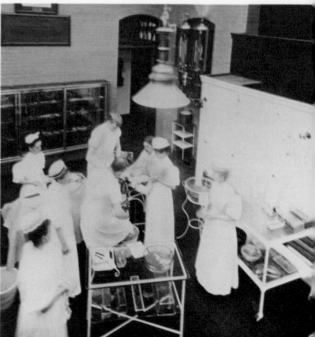

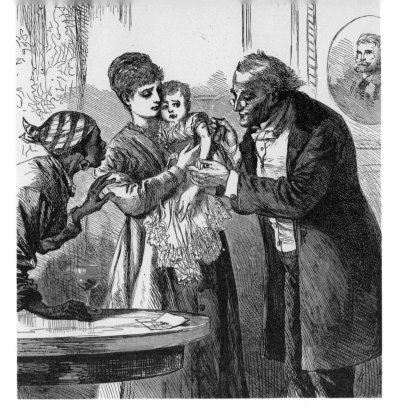

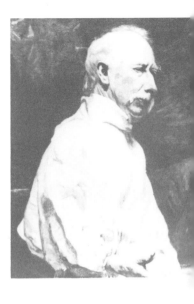

Left: Vaccinating the Baby. Illustration, c. 1870. [L.C.] For many years medicine was practiced more often than not in the patient's home rather than the doctor's office. *Right:* Dr. D. Hayes Agnew. Detail from painting by Thomas Eakins, "The Agnew Clinic," 1889. [L.C.] A noted surgeon, Dr. Agnew was one of the first to use asepsis in the operating room. *Below:* Surgical Scene in a Home. Photograph, late 19th century. [N.L.M.] Anesthesia is being administered with the assistance of nurses.

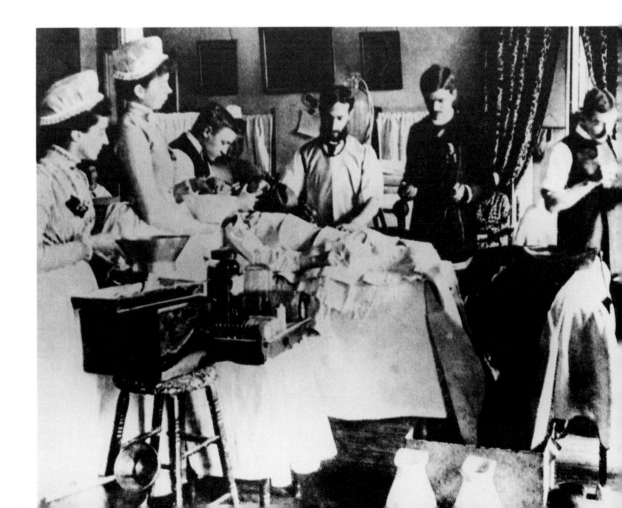

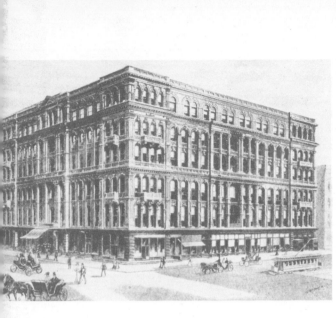

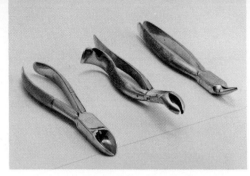

Left: Northwestern University Building. Photograph, late 19th century. [N.M.H.T.] The Dental School occupied the top three floors when Dr. Black became its dean.
Above: Dental Instruments. Metal, late 19th century. [E.L.]

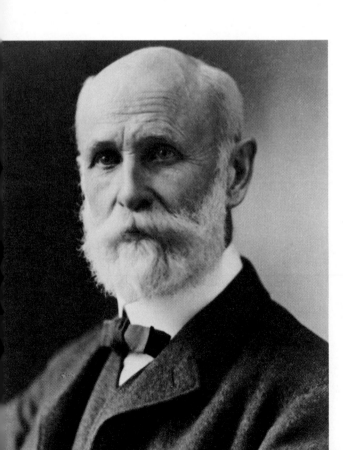

Above: Dental chair and Foot-Operated Pneumatic Drill. Mixed materials, late 19th century. [N.L.M.] *Left:* Dr. Greene Vardiman Black. Photograph, c. 1898. [N.M.H.T.] Because of his many contributions to dental surgery and dental education, Dr. Black (1836-1915), was known as "The Father of American Dentistry."

Right: Nurses Training to be Surgical Assistants. Photograph, c. 1899. [M.C.N.Y.] By 1899 these nursing students at St. Luke's Hospital, New York City, were being taught antiseptic procedures—the use of surgical gloves, sterile instruments, etc.—for which they were increasingly responsible, and to assist in surgery. *Below:* Scene in a Bellevue Ward. Engraving, c. 1885. [F.L.I.] The first modern nurses' training school in the United States was established at Bellevue Hospital, New York City in 1873. *Below right:* Nurses with Lanterns. Photograph, 1899. [N.L.M.] These nurses, assigned to the night shift at Yale-New Haven Hospital in New Haven, Connecticut, posed for a portrait before making their appointed rounds.

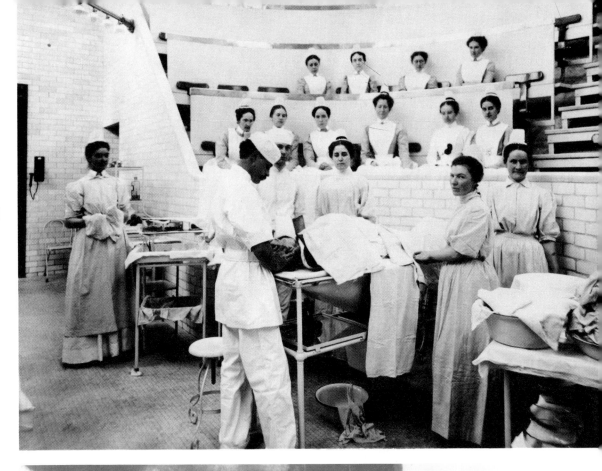

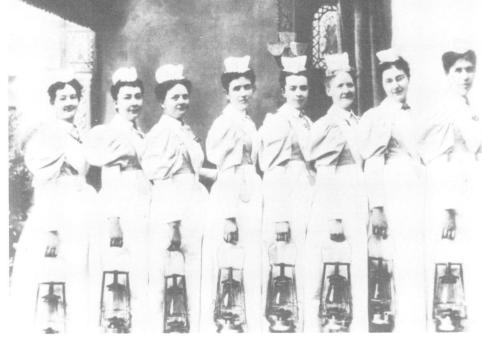

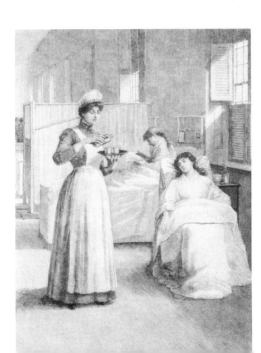

Right: Title Page: *Richardson & Co., Importers and Wholesale Druggists.* Print, 1880. [E.L.C.] The following is a collection of facsimile pages from the Cost and Stock Book, or catalogue, issued by a leading wholesaler to its retail pharmacy customers. Richardson & Co. of St. Louis offered a broad and varied range of merchandise.

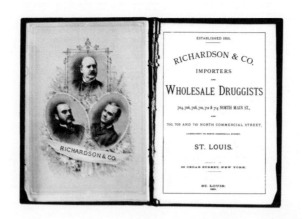

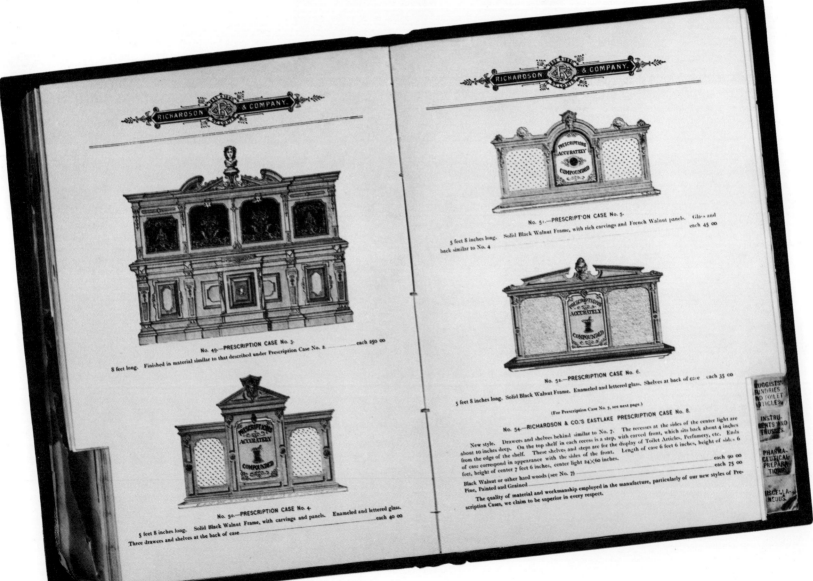

No. 49.—PRESCRIPTION CASE No. 3. each 250 00

8 feet long. Finished in material similar to that described under Prescription Case No. 2.

No. 50.—PRESCRIPTION CASE No. 4.

5 feet 8 inches long. Solid Black Walnut Frame, with carvings and panels. Enameled and lettered glass. Three drawers and shelves at the back of case. each 40 00

No. 51.—PRESCRIPTION CASE No. 5. each 45 00

5 feet 8 inches long. Solid Black Walnut Frame, with rich carvings and French Walnut panels. Glass and back similar to No. 4.

No. 52.—PRESCRIPTION CASE No. 6. each 35 00

5 feet 8 inches long. Solid Black Walnut Frame. Enameled and lettered glass. Shelves at back of case.

(For Prescription Case No. 7, see next page.)

No. 54.—RICHARDSON & CO.'S EASTLAKE PRESCRIPTION CASE No. 8.

New style. Drawers and shelves behind similar to No. 7. The recesses at the sides of the center light are about 10 inches deep. On the top shelf in each recess is a step, with carved front, which sits back about 4 inches from the edge of the shelf. These shelves and steps are for the display of Toilet Articles, Perfumery, etc. Ends of case correspond in appearance with the sides of the front. Length of case 6 feet 6 inches, height of sides 6 feet, height of center 7 feet 6 inches, center light 24×60 inches.

Black Walnut or other hard woods (see No. 7) each 90 00
Pine, Painted and Grained each 75 00

The quality of material and workmanship employed in the manufacture, particularly of our new styles of Prescription Cases, we claim to be superior in every respect.

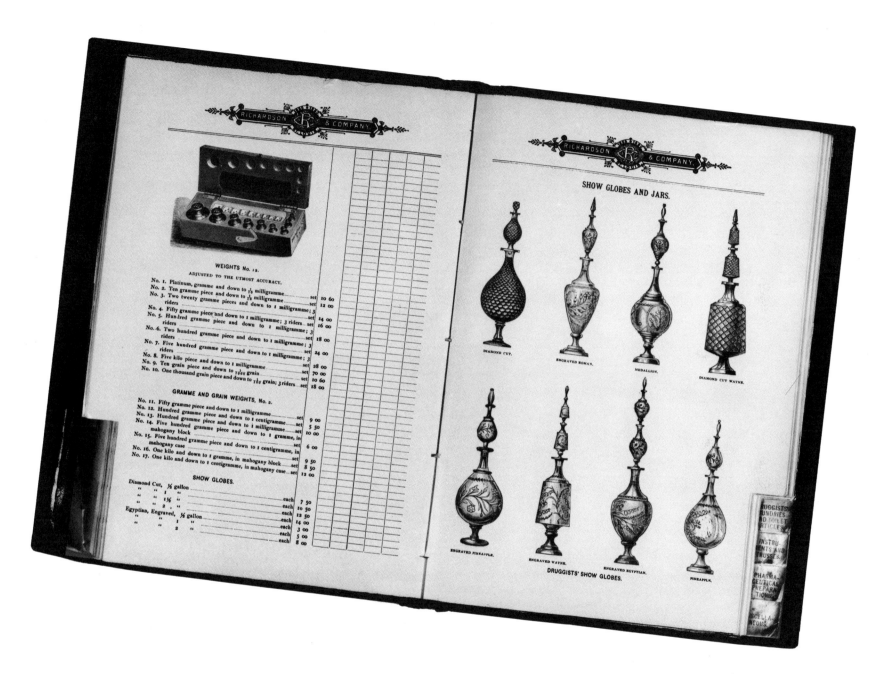

WEIGHTS No. 12.

ADJUSTED TO THE UTMOST ACCURACY.

No. 1. Platinum, gramme and down to 1/10 milligramme
No. 2. Ten gramme piece and down to 1/10 milligramme............set 10 60
No. 3. Two twenty gramme pieces and down to 1 milligramme.....set 12 00
riders
No. 4. Fifty gramme piece and down to 1 milligramme; 3 riders....set 14 00
No. 5. Hundred gramme piece and down to 1 milligramme............set 16 00
riders
No. 6. Two hundred gramme piece and down to 1 milligramme; 3
riders ....set 18 00
No. 7. Five hundred gramme piece and down to 1 milligramme; 3
riders ....set 24 00
No. 8. Five kilo piece and down to 1 milligramme
No. 9. Ten grain piece and down to 1/1000 grain.....................set 28 00
No. 10. One thousand grain piece and down to 1/10 grain; 3 riders..set 70 00
set 10 60
set 18 00

GRAMME AND GRAIN WEIGHTS, No. 2.

No. 11. Fifty gramme piece and down to 1 milligramme
No. 12. Hundred gramme piece and down to 1 milligramme...........set 9 00
No. 13. Hundred gramme piece and down to 1 centigramme..........set 5 50
No. 14. Five hundred gramme piece and down to 1 gramme, in
mahogany block ....set 10 00
No. 15. Five hundred gramme piece and down to 1 centigramme, in
mahogany case ....set 6 00
No. 16. One kilo and down to 1 gramme, in mahogany block........set 9 50
No. 17. One kilo and down to 1 centigramme, in mahogany case....set 12 00

SHOW GLOBES.

Diamond Cut, 1/2 gallon
"   1   " ....each 7 50
"   1 1/2 " ....each 10 50
"   2   " ....each 12 50
Egyptian, Engraved, 1/2 gallon ....each 14 00
"   1   " ....each 3 00
"   2   " ....each 5 00
each 8 00

SHOW GLOBES AND JARS.

DIAMOND CUT.   ENGRAVED ROMAN.   MEDALLION.   DIAMOND CUT WAYNE.

ENGRAVED PINEAPPLE.   ENGRAVED WAYNE.   ENGRAVED EGYPTIAN.   PINEAPPLE.

DRUGGISTS' SHOW GLOBES.

Shown here are display fixtures, measuring weights and show globes. The catalogue also offered compounding and pill-making equipment, paints and brushes, soaps, perfumes, liquors, lard and oil, stationery, doctors' and dentists' instruments, and imported and American patent medicines.

The Richardson firm also offered the products of the growing number of responsible American ethical drug houses. Shown are listings for Allaire Woodward and Co. and Eli Lilly. Others included: McKesson and Robbins, W. S. Merrell and Co., Parke, Davis and Co., Richardson and Co., E. R. Squibb, and W. R. Warner and Co.

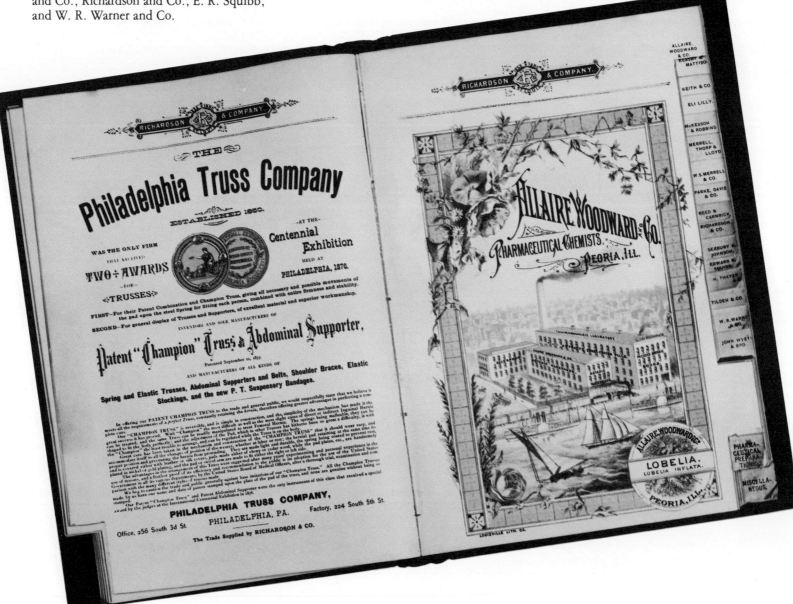

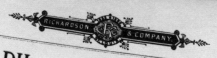

PIL. APHRODISIACA
(LILLY).
Or, Pil. Damiana cum Phosphori et Nucis Vomicæ.

℞ Extract Damiana . . . .
Phosphorus . . . . 2 grs.
Ext. Nux Vomica . . . . ⅒ gr.
⅒ gr.

DOSE—One to three Pills three times daily with food.

"DAMIANA is, beyond a doubt, the most reliable, useful and permanent tonic to the genital organs of both sexes known; acting, as it does, directly upon the nervous system, it restores, as it were, the debilitated functions of the princip'l organs of the human frame, and is unsurpassed as a nervine. Its merits are now established as a powerful, permanent and determined aphrodisiac, as well as an alterative aperient of remarkably fine quality."— JOHN J. CALDWELL, M. D., IN NEW YORK MEDICAL RECORD, Nov. 3, 1877, page 694.

PHOSPHORUS and NUX VOMICA, as is well known to the profession, act as nutritive tonics to the nervous system, especially the spinal cord, and can be relied upon as possessing real aphrodisiac power. The excellent results so frequently reported as following the use of my FLUID EXTRACT OF DAMIANA in connection with my PILLS of PHOSPHORUS, and PHOSPHORUS with NUX VOMICA, has induced me to combine these valuable remedial agents in the pill form, thus overcoming all objections to their separate use. As the DAMIANA used is the genuine TURNERA APHRODISIACA, the preparation can be relied upon. By my process for the manufacture of PHOSPHORUS PILLS, thorough sub-division of Phosphorus in the mass is obtained, and, with a coating perfectly PROTECTING it from OXIDATION, there is nothing further to be desired. It is necessary that the administration of this pill be continued from THREE TO FOUR WEEKS, or until the SYSTEM IS THOROUGHLY UNDER THE INFLUENCE OF THE REMEDY. Caution should be taken in its use as in other combinations of Phosphorus, and should not be taken in any case except when prescribed by a physician. It is indicated in MENTAL OVER-WORK, SEXUAL DEBILITY, IMPOTENCY. It is decidedly beneficial in cases of NOCTURNAL EMISSIONS, the result of excesses, MENTAL APATHY, or indifference, and in an ENFEEBLED CONDITION OF THE GENERAL SYSTEM, with WEAKNESS or DULL PAIN IN THE LUMBO-SACRAL REGION. In diseases of the REPRODUCTIVE ORGANS of the female, and especially of the uterus, it is one of our most valuable agents, acting as a UTERINE TONIC, and gradually removing abnormal conditions, while, at the same time, it imparts tone and vigor; hence, it is of value in LEUCORRHŒA, AMENORRHŒA, DYSMENORRHŒA, and to remove the tendency to repeated miscarriages.

CAUTION.

The steady and increasing demand for PIL. APHRODISIACA, since introduced by me three years ago, has induced imitations, in one instance at least substituting the drug Damiana for the solid extract. In order to get the original and best preparation, "PIL. APHRODISIACA (LILLY)" should always be written on orders or prescriptions.

For Sale by RICHARDSON & CO.

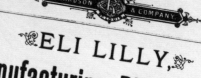

ELI LILLY,
Manufacturing Pharmacist,

36 and 38 South Meridian St.,

INDIANAPOLIS, IND.

"PERFECTION"
GELATINE COATED PILLS.

CONTINUOUS COATING of PURE GELATINE, impervious to the air, and much superior to the old needle process.

SUGAR COATED PILLS.

In UNIFORMITY OF SIZE and SHAPE, BEAUTY OF FINISH and PRECISION to FORMULA they are UNEXCELLED.

FLUID EXTRACTS.

From BEST SELECTED DRUGS, by my IMPROVED COLD PROCESS.

ELIXIRS, SYRUPS, WINES,
SACCHARATED PEPSINE,
AROMAT. LIQUID PEPSINE.

ALL GOODS SOLD UNDER ABSOLUTE GUARANTEE OF QUALITY.

For Sale by RICHARDSON & CO.

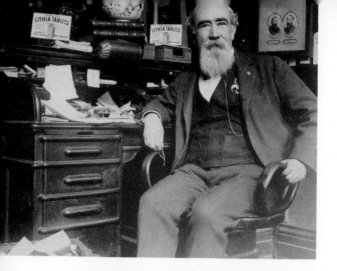

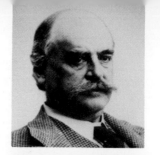

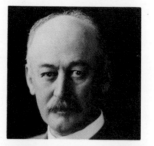

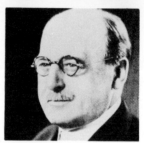

Left: William R. Warner. Photograph, c. 1880s. [W.L.C.] Mr. Warner, who was one of the first to coat pills with sugar, founded the William R. Warner Company not long after graduating from Philadelphia's College of Pharmacy and Science in 1856. By 1876, the company occupied a six-story building in the city and grew to be one of America's leading pharmaceutical manufacturers.

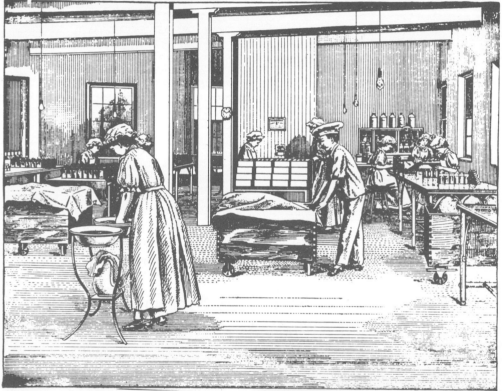

Above, top to bottom: Robert Wood Johnson, James Wood Johnson, Edward Mead Johnson. Photographs, late 19th century. [J.J. & M.J.] The three brothers founded Johnson and Johnson. *Left:* One of the Aseptic Rooms, Johnson and Johnson Laboratories. Print, c. 1890. [J.J.] *Below, near left:* Worker Packing Sterile Gauze. Photograph, c. 1892. [J.J.] Johnson and Johnson quickly recognized the importance of Dr. Lister's principle of antiseptics in surgery. *Below, far left:* Advertisement for Zonweiss Toothpaste, June 1887. [J.J.] With the appearance of Zonweiss, Johnson and Johnson introduced ready-made toothpaste in a tube.

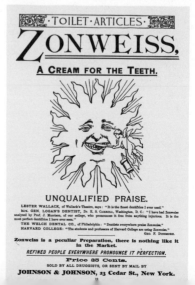

· TOILET · ARTICLES ·

ZONWEISS,

A CREAM FOR THE TEETH.

UNQUALIFIED PRAISE.

LESTER WALLACK, of Wallack's Theatre, says: "It is the finest dentifrice I ever used."

hrs. GEN. LOGAN'S DENTIST, Dr. E. S. CARROLL, Washington, D. C.: "I have had Zonweiss analyzed by Prof. J. Morrison, of our college, who pronounces it free from anything injurious. It is the most perfect dentifrice I have ever seen."

THE WELCH DENTAL CO., of Philadelphia: "Dentists everywhere praise Zonweiss."

HARVARD COLLEGE: "The students and professors of Harvard College are using Zonweiss."
GEO. F. DINSMORE.

Zonweiss is a peculiar Preparation, there is nothing like it in the Market.

REFINED PEOPLE EVERYWHERE PRONOUNCE IT PERFECTION.

Price 35 Cents.

SOLD BY ALL DRUGGISTS, OR SENT BY MAIL BY

JOHNSON & JOHNSON, 23 Cedar St., New York.

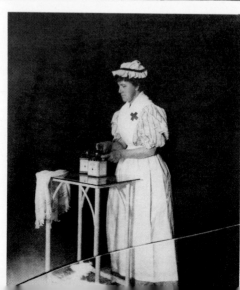

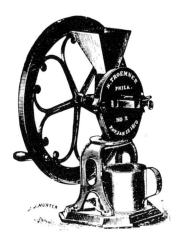

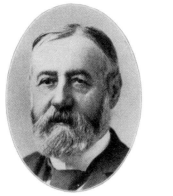
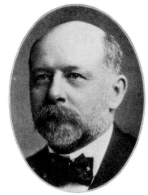

Above: Drug Mill. Metal, late 19th century. [P.C.] *Above, near right:* Mahlon K. Smith. Photograph, c. 1880. *Above, far right:* Mahlon N. Kline. Photograph, c. 1880. [Both: S.K.C.] The distinguished pharmaceutical company SmithKline Corporation traces its roots back to 1830, when John K. Smith opened a pharmacy in Philadelphia. In the last quarter of the 19th century the company was led by the key partners shown here. *Right:* Dr. Fitch's Prescription Scale. Metal, late 19th century. [H.M.M.] Patented in 1885, this pocket scale used by pharmacists and physicians was made by N.V. Randolph & Co., Richmond, Va.

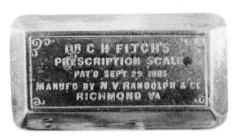

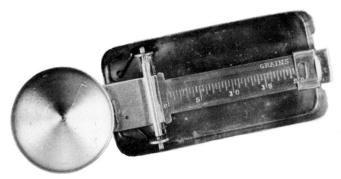

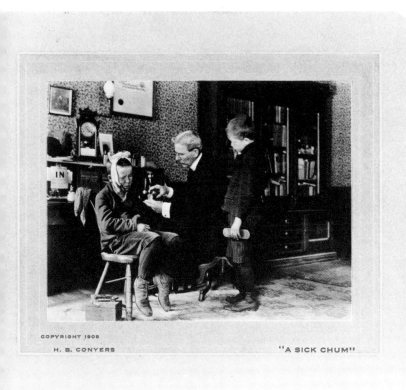

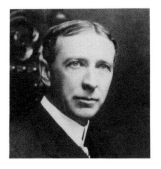
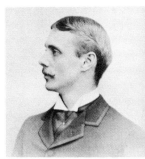

Above left: William McLaren Bristol; *right:* John Ripley Myers. Photographs, late 19th century. [B.M.] Messrs. Bristol and Myers founded their Clinton, N.Y. pharmaceutical house as The Clinton Pharmaceutical Co., incorporating as Bristol-Myers Company in 1900. *Left:* "A Sick Chum." Photograph, c. 1900. [L.C.] A turn-of-the-century doctor administers medicine to a young shoeshine boy.

95

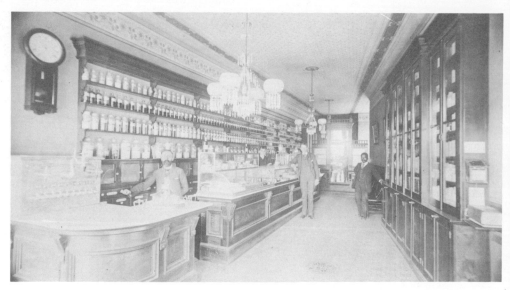

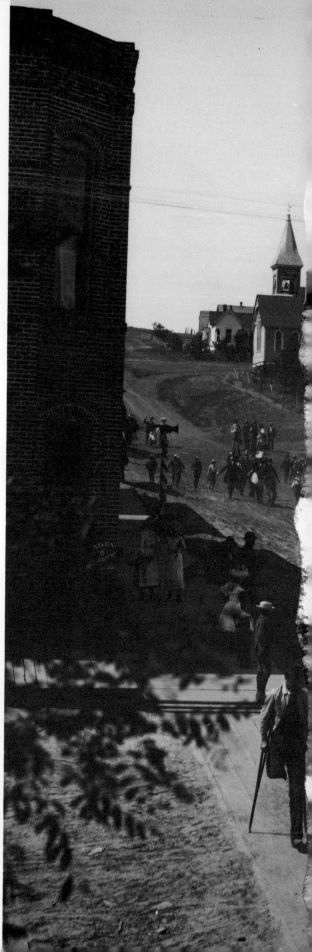

Above: Castoria Pharmacy, Baltimore, Maryland. Photograph, late 19th century. [A.P.A.] *Below left:* A Chinese Drugstore. Engraving, 1899. [N.L.M.] This San Francisco Chinese pharmacy maintained a stock of herbs and medicines of the ancient Chinese pharmacopoeia. *Below right:* Asa G. Candler's Pharmacy. Photograph, c. 1890. [M.9.] Asa G. Candler, a partner in this Atlanta pharmacy, bought the rights to Coca-Cola from chemist John Pemberton, who originated the formula in 1886. Initially it was marketed as a medicine.

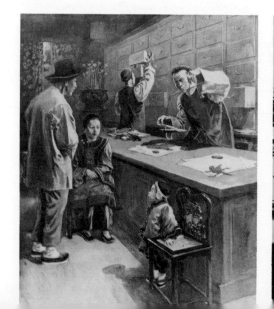

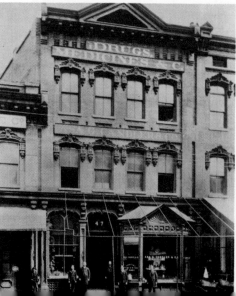

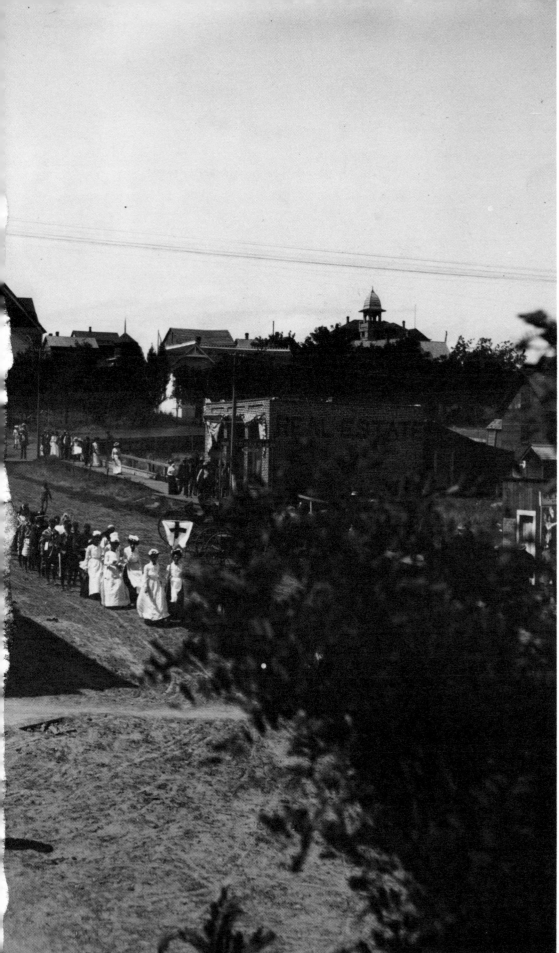

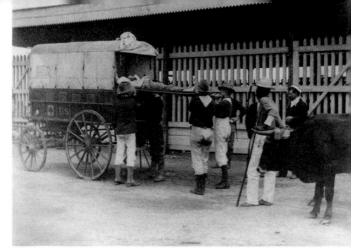

Left: Red Cross Parade during Spanish-American War. Photograph, c. 1898.[M.11.] A small town's patriotic mood was captured by photographer W.A. Raymond. *Above:* Unloading Spanish-American War Wounded. Photograph, 1898. [N.L.M.] An American casualty of the fighting in Cuba is removed from an ambulance at the port of Mayaguez for transport back to the U.S. on the Hospital Ship *Relief. Below:* H.S. *Relief.* Photograph, 1898. [N.L.M.]

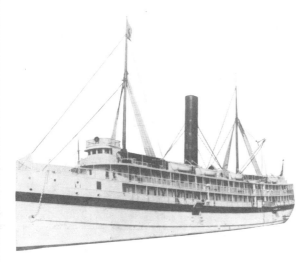

97

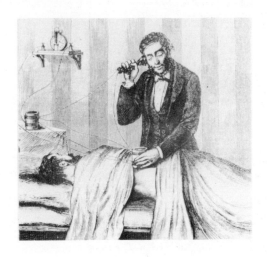

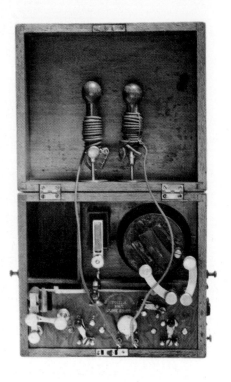

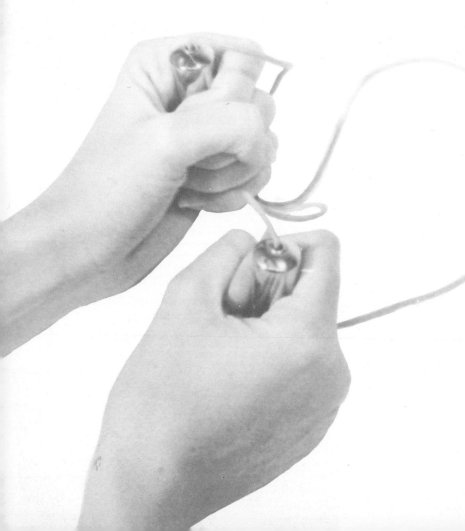

Above left: A Device for Locating Fragments in Wounds. Engraving, 1881. [P.C.] *Above right:* The Fleming Battery. Mixed materials, 1865. [H.M.S.] *Left:* Household Coil. Mixed materials, late 19th century. [H.M.M.] From Benjamin Franklin's time electrotherapy had many adherents in America. Among other things, electricity was thought to have curative power for consumption, palsy, venereal disease, cancer, blindness, and worms.

Right: Electrostatic Machine and Patient.
Photograph, late 19th century. [H.M.P.S.]
Mobile photographer William Wilson,
probably hired to record the machine, posed
a ''patient'' disguised by a Mardi Gras mask.
Below left: Moorhead's Magnetic Machines.
Advertisement, late 19th century. [L.C.] A
household coil is seen being utilized in a
fancy Victorian parlor. *Below right:* Early
EKG Machine. Mixed materials, late 19th-
early 20th century. [P.C.P.S.] In the early
1900s, William Einthoven introduced the
first practical device for recording the heart's
behavior, the string galvanometer, an
invaluable contribution to the harnessing of
electricity for medical purposes.

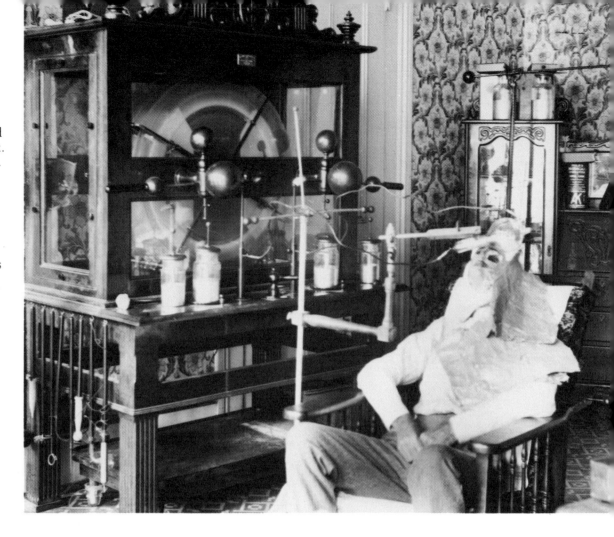

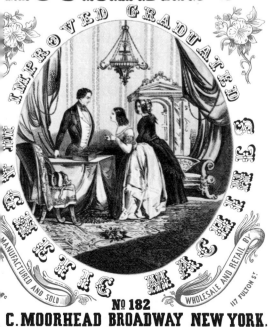

MOORHEAD'S

No 182
C. MOORHEAD BROADWAY NEW YORK.

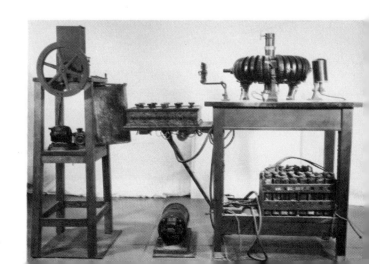

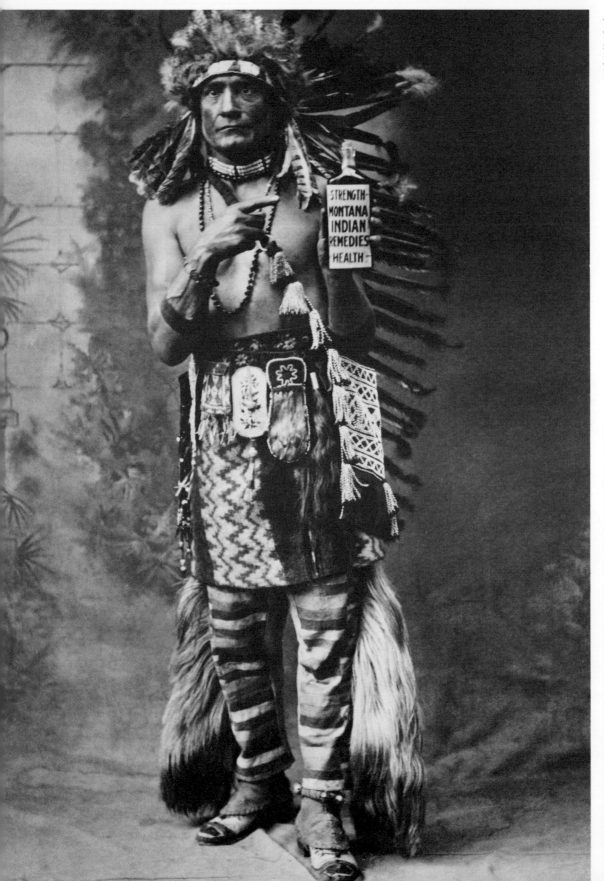

Left: Indian as Pitchman. Photograph, 19th century. [L.C.] A Native American posed for a studio shot for Montana Indian Remedies.
Below: Kickapoo Indian Medicine Show at Marine, Minn. Photograph, c. 1890. [M.H.S.]

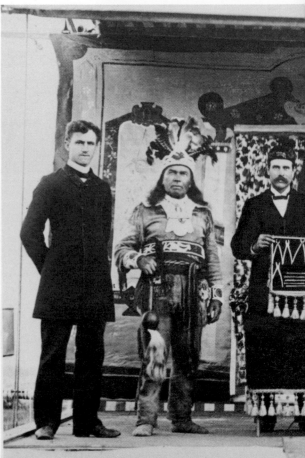

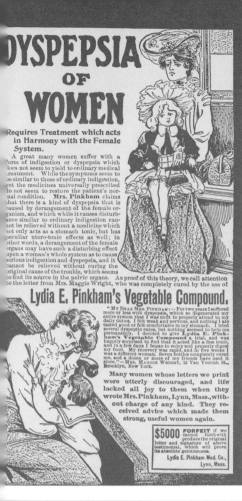

DYSPEPSIA OF WOMEN

Requires Treatment which acts in Harmony with the Female System.

A great many women suffer with a form of indigestion or dyspepsia which does not seem to yield to ordinary medical treatment. While the symptoms seem to be similar to those of ordinary indigestion, yet the medicines universally prescribed do not seem to restore the patient's normal condition. Mrs. Pinkham claims that there is a kind of dyspepsia that is caused by derangement of the female organism, and which while it causes disturbance similar to ordinary indigestion cannot be relieved without a medicine which not only acts as a stomach tonic, but has peculiar utero-tonic effects as well; in other words, a derangement of the female organs may have such a disturbing effect upon a woman's whole system as to cause serious indigestion and dyspepsia, and it cannot be relieved without curing the original cause of the trouble, which seems to find its source in the pelvic organs. As proof of this theory, we call attention to the letter from Mrs. Maggie Wright, who was completely cured by the use of

Lydia E. Pinkham's Vegetable Compound.

"MY DEAR MRS. PINKHAM:— For two years I suffered more or less with dyspepsia, which so degenerated my entire system that I was unfit to properly attend to my daily duties. I felt weak and nervous, and nothing I ate tasted good or felt comfortable in my stomach. I tried several dyspepsia cures, but nothing seemed to help me permanently. I decided to give Lydia E. Pinkham's Vegetable Compound a trial, and was happily surprised to find that it acted like a fine tonic, and in a few days I began to enjoy and properly digest my food. My recovery was rapid, and in five weeks I was a different woman. Seven bottles completely cured me, and a dozen or more of my friends have used it since."— MRS. MAGGIE WRIGHT, 12 Van Voorhis St., Brooklyn, New York.

Many women whose letters we print were utterly discouraged, and life lacked all joy to them when they wrote Mrs. Pinkham, Lynn, Mass., without charge of any kind. They received advice which made them strong, useful women again.

$5000 FORFEIT if we cannot forthwith produce the original letter and signature of above testimonial, which will prove its absolute genuineness.
Lydia E. Pinkham Med. Co., Lynn, Mass.

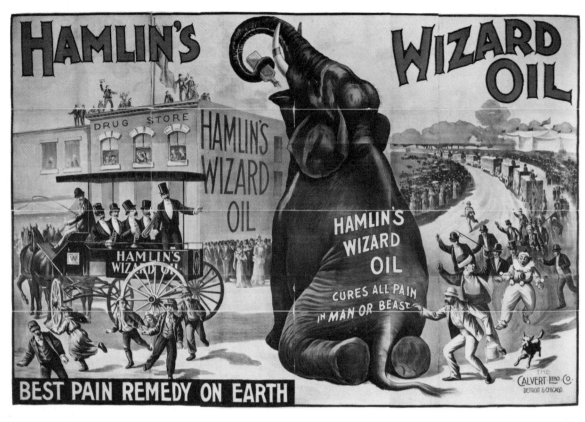

HAMLIN'S WIZARD OIL

DRUG STORE
HAMLIN'S WIZARD OIL
HAMLIN'S WIZARD OIL
HAMLIN'S WIZARD OIL CURES ALL PAIN IN MAN OR BEAST
THE CALVERT LITHO. CO. DETROIT & CHICAGO

BEST PAIN REMEDY ON EARTH

Above left: Lydia E. Pinkham's Vegetable Compound Advertisement. Print, c. 1900. [F.L.I.] There were many successful manufacturers of proprietary medicines, but Lydia E. Pinkham of Lynn, Mass. became a legend. *Above and below right:* Patent Medicine Advertisements. Prints, 19th century. [L.C.]

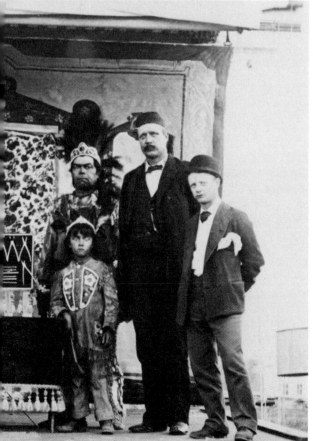

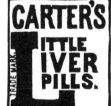

SICK HEADACHE

CARTER'S LITTLE LIVER PILLS.

TRADE MARK

Positively Cured by these Little Pills.

They also relieve Distress from Dyspepsia, Indigestion and Too Hearty Eating. A perfect remedy for Dizziness, Nausea, Drowsiness, Bad Taste in the Mouth, Coated Tongue, Pain in the Side, &c. They regulate the Bowels and prevent Constipation and Piles. The smallest and easiest to take. Only one pill a dose. Purely Vegetable.

CARTER MEDICINE CO., Prop'rs, New York.

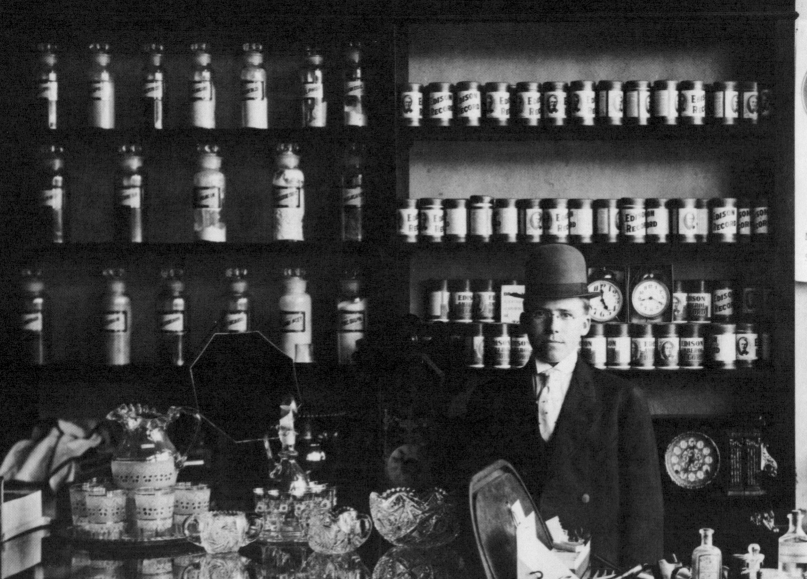

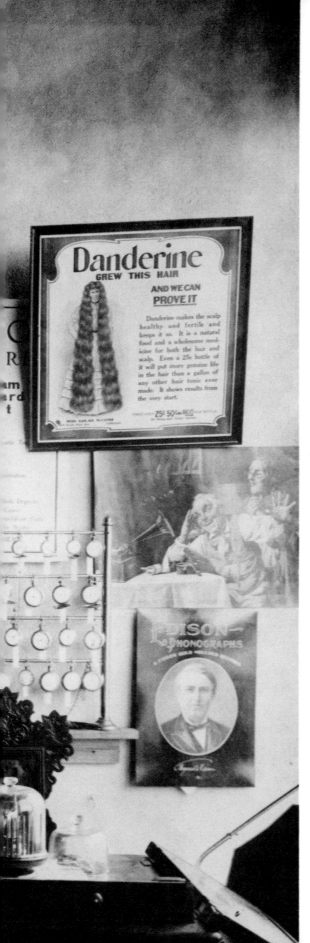

CHAPTER SIX

1900-1909

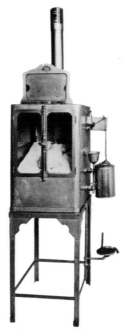

As this advertisement from *Hostetter's United States Almanac* (1867) indicates, patent medicines or nostrums could cure just about anything.

"Dread Diarhhea, that cannot be
Cured by destructive Mercury;
Slow constitutional decay,
That brings death nearer, day by day;
Nervous prostration, mental gloom,
Heralds of madness or the tomb;
For these, though Mineral nostrums fail,
Means of relief at last we hail,
HOSTETTER'S BITTERS—medicine sure,
Not to *prevent,* alone, but cure."

Throughout the 19th century, such fraudulent claims played on the population's ignorance. The exotic nature of the advertised cures held far more allure than physicians' habitual bleedings and purgings.

With the founding of The Philadelphia College of Pharmacy in 1821, the American Pharmaceutical Association in 1852, and pharmaceutical companies, serious efforts began to improve the quality of drugs and the standards of the pharmacists' profession. Primary support came with passage of the Pure Food and Drug Act of 1906, a major turning point in pharmaceutical history.

Left: Silvernail Drugstore. Photograph, c. 1910 [M.H.S.] The name of this earnest young druggist in Marietta, Minnesota is unknown. *Above:* Baby in Incubator. Photograph, c. 1900. [M.C.N.Y.] At the turn of the century, New York's Sloane Maternity Hospital was equipped with an electric-powered incubator for premature infants.

103

1900: 75,994,575 inhabitants; 39.7% urban, 60.3% rural
McKinley elected President
Carry Nation began anti-saloon campaign

1901: McKinley assassinated; Theodore Roosevelt successor

1902: Congress authorized Panama Canal
1902-32 Oliver Wendell Holmes, Justice of Supreme Court

1903: Department of Commerce & Labor created
First direct primary voting, Wisconsin
Wright Brothers first heavier-than-air flight

1904: Roosevelt elected President
1904-14: Construction of Panama Canal

1900

1900: The American Association of Pathologists and Bacteriologists was founded.

1900: Walter Reed (1851-1902), went to Havana to investigate yellow fever among American soldiers in Cuba. Reed and his co-workers used human volunteers to prove the earlier theory of Carlos Finlay (1833-1915), that the mosquito was the carrier. William Gorgas (1854-1920), the U.S. Army's chief sanitary officer in Cuba, directed a three-month mosquito-extermination campaign that eliminated the insects and the fever from Havana.

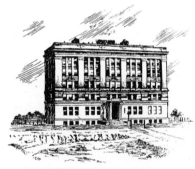

The Rockefeller Institute for Medical Research

1900: Red blood cells were divided into three blood groups by Karl Landsteiner. His discovery made blood transfusion a reliable lifesaving procedure rather than a risky experiment. In 1930 he became the first American citizen to receive the Nobel Prize in medicine, and in 1940 he discovered the Rh factor, of vital importance in obstetrics.

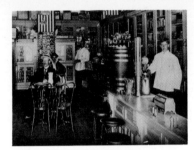

Turn of the Century Pharmacy

1901: A Riva-Rocci sphygmomanometer, the first practical apparatus for measuring blood pressure, was brought to Baltimore from Italy by surgeon Harvey Cushing (1869-1939). Cushing introduced the sphygmomanometer to American medicine and stressed the importance of using it at regular intervals during surgery.

1901: Rockefeller Institute for Medical Research was established in New York City. The first American institute devoted wholly to medical research, and funded by John D. Rockefeller, Sr., initially granted money just to existing laboratories—about $12,000 in 1901. Its own laboratory opened in 1906, its hospital in 1910.

1902: The Marine Hospital Service expanded its responsibilities and became the Public Health and Marine Hospital Service. A Hygienic Laboratory was established in Washington, D.C., to undertake research and to regulate the interstate sale of serums, toxins and other products.

1902: The first U.S. laboratory for scientific research built by a commercial company was erected by Parke, Davis & Company. In 1903, License No. 1 for "the manufacture of viruses, toxins, serums, and other analogous products" was issued to Parke, Davis by the U.S. Treasury Department.

1902: The Peter Bent Brigham Hospital in Boston was incorporated, funded by the $1.3 million fortune left by Brigham in 1877 to endow "a hospital for the care of sick persons in indigent circumstances." The hospital was built ten years later next to Harvard Medical School, and for the first time, the University was given a decisive vote in the hiring of hospital medical staff.

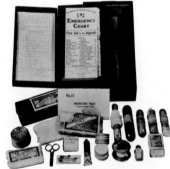

The First Aid Department of the Red Cross was Formed in 1903

1903: The American Society of Clinical Surgeons was organized.

1903: The first full-time school nurse, Lina Rogers, was appointed in New York City.

1904: The Association for the Study and Prevention of Tuberculosis was founded. In 1918 it became the National Tuberculosis Association and 55 years later, the American Lung Association. This was the first voluntary health organization to have a major impact upon public health and health legislation. By 1917 each state and territory had its own tuberculosis society.

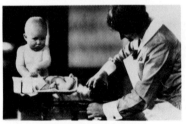

Nurse Weighing Infant

1905: The American Child Health Association was formed. In the same year, the American Social Hygiene Association was established.

1905: Harvey Cushing, neurosurgeon, took charge of the new Hunterian Laboratory of Experimental Medicine at Johns Hopkins. He carried out experiments in surgery of the pituitary gland. Later associated with Harvard (1912-1932) and Yale (1933-1937), Cushing was noted as a teacher and author as well as for his contributions to brain surgery. He established the use of local rather than general anesthesia for brain operations, and pioneered the use of radiographs and blood-pressure readings in diagnosis.

1905: Industrial Workers of the World formed

1906: Pure Food & Drug Act; Meat Inspection Act became law
San Francisco earthquake and fire

1907: Record 1,285,349 emigrate to U.S.
Oklahoma became 46th state
1907-09: Six states enacted "dry" laws

1908: Ford introduced Model T
William Howard Taft elected President

1909: Admiral Peary reached North Pole
National Association for the Advancement of Colored People founded

1905: One of the last epidemics of yellow fever in the United States occurred in New Orleans.

1905: High-school education, four years of medical school, and a year's internship were recommended by the A.M.A.'s Council on Medical Education as the "ideal standard."

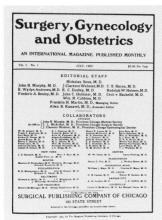

Magazine Cover

1905: The first American journal for surgeons, *Surgery, Gynecology and Obstetrics,* began publication.

1906: Alexis Carrel (1873-1944), French-American surgeon, joined the Rockefeller Institute. For his dramatic experiments in the transplant and replacement of living organs and blood vessels, he received the 1912 Nobel Prize. In 1936, with Charles A. Lindbergh, he invented the first artificial or mechanical heart.

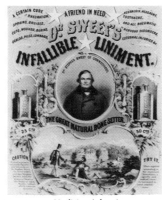

Patent Medicine Advertisement

1906: The first federal Food and Drug Act was passed during the reform administration of Theodore Roosevelt. This reduced the deceptive practices of the 19th century, and was the first federal legislation to protect the buyers of medicinal drugs. Harvey Washington Wiley, Indiana-born chief chemist of the Department of Agriculture, was largely responsible for the act's passage and administration.

1907: The first Christmas Seals were sold to raise funds to combat tuberculosis. The idea, conceived in Denmark, was introduced by the journalist and social reformer Jacob A. Riis (1849-1914). Sales raised $3,000.

1907: The Association of Hospital Superintendents was renamed the American Hospital Association of the United States and Canada.

1907: The use of toxin-antitoxin in diphtheria was suggested by Theobald Smith (1859-1934), noted professor of comparative pathology at Harvard, and director of the department of animal pathology at Rockefeller Institute.

1907: The study of nutrition and metabolism was advanced by construction of a calorimeter that could measure heat production, oxygen consumption and the elimination of carbon dioxide. The basal metabolism of normal individuals could be determined, and the effect of diseases on the metabolic rate could be measured.

1907: Howard Taylor Ricketts, a young pathologist, proved that Rocky Mountain Spotted Fever is transmitted from animals to humans by infected ticks. The small disease-causing bacteria were named Rickettsia. In 1910 Ricketts died of typhus in Mexico City, while proving the fever was also transmitted by lice.

1908: Chicago was the first major city to require pasteurization of milk.

1908: Clifford Whittingham Beers (1876-1943), a young businessman who became the founder of the American mental hygiene movement, published his autobiographical account of confinement in an unsympathetic mental institution, *A Mind That Found Itself.*

1908: Maude Abbott, a pathologist whose classification of congenital heart defects was a major stepping stone to cardiac surgery later in the 20th century, published her studies on *Congenital Malformations of The Heart.*

1909: Psychoanalysis first received public recognition when Sigmund Freud (1856-1939), and Carl Jung (1875-1961), gave a series of lectures at Clark University, Worcester, Massachusetts.

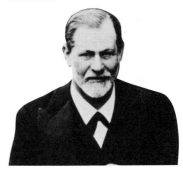

Sigmund Freud

1909: The National Committee for Mental Hygiene was established, largely as a result of the work of Clifford W. Beers. After its formation, the care of psychiatric patients improved greatly.

1909: The Society of Biology and Medicine was organized.

1909: Soldiers and officers of the U.S. Army were vaccinated against typhoid fever.

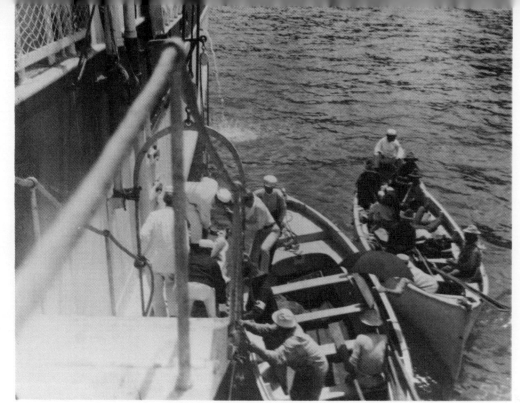

Right: Yellow Fever Victims Being Taken Aboard Hospital Ship *Relief* off Cuba. Photograph, c. 1900. [N.L.M.] *Below:* Dr. Walter Reed. Photograph, c. 1900. [N.L.M.] *Below right:* General William C. Gorgas. Photograph, c. 1904-14. [N.L.M.] Following Reed's findings, General Gorgas, also of the Army Medical Corps, instituted anti-mosquito sanitation measures in the Panama Canal Zone that permitted the construction of the canal.

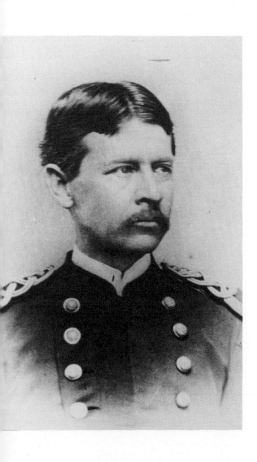

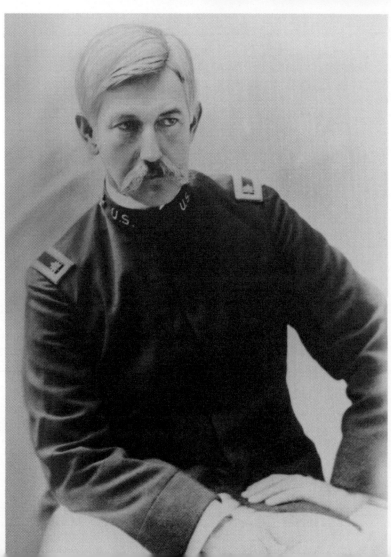

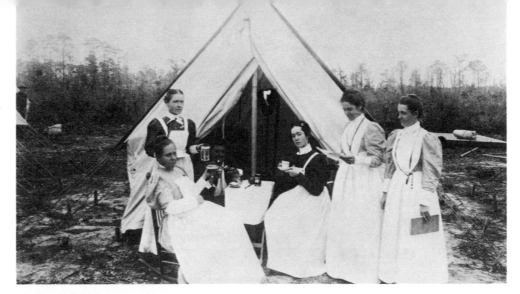

Right: Leisure Hours in Camp. Photograph, c. 1900. [N.L.M.] Six nurses are seen on a tea or coffee break at a fever quarantine camp in the Southeastern U.S. *Below:* Yellow Fever Campaign, New Orleans. Photograph, c. 1900. [N.L.M.] One of the last yellow fever epidemics in the U.S. struck New Orleans in 1905. Shown, posed with Governor Blanchard of Louisiana, are U.S. Public Health officers who served in the state.

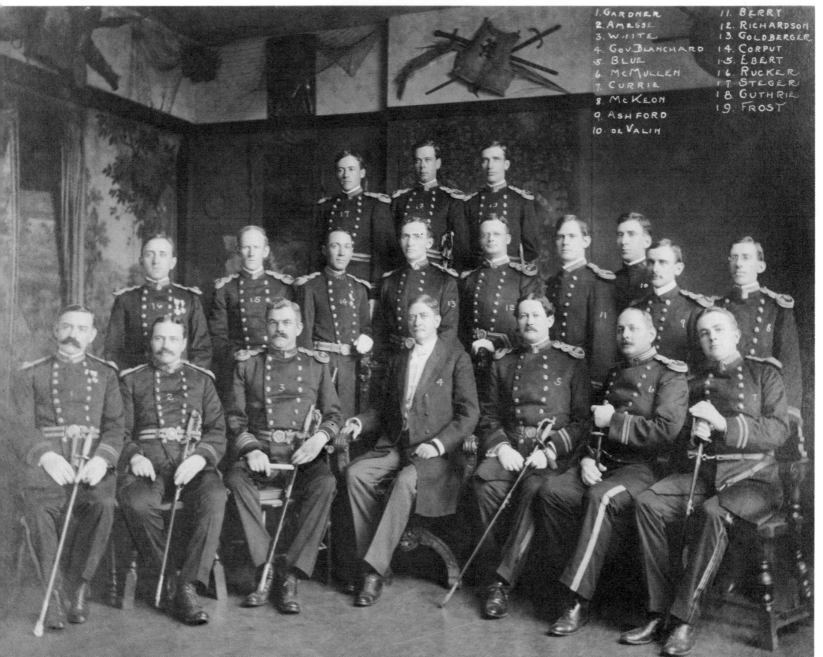

1. GARDNER
2. AMESSE
3. WHITE
4. GOV BLANCHARD
5. BLUE
6. McMULLEN
7. CURRIE
8. McKEON
9. ASHFORD
10. DE VALIN
11. BERRY
12. RICHARDSON
13. GOLDBERGER
14. CORPUT
15. EBERT
16. RUCKER
17. STEGER
18. GUTHRIE
19. FROST

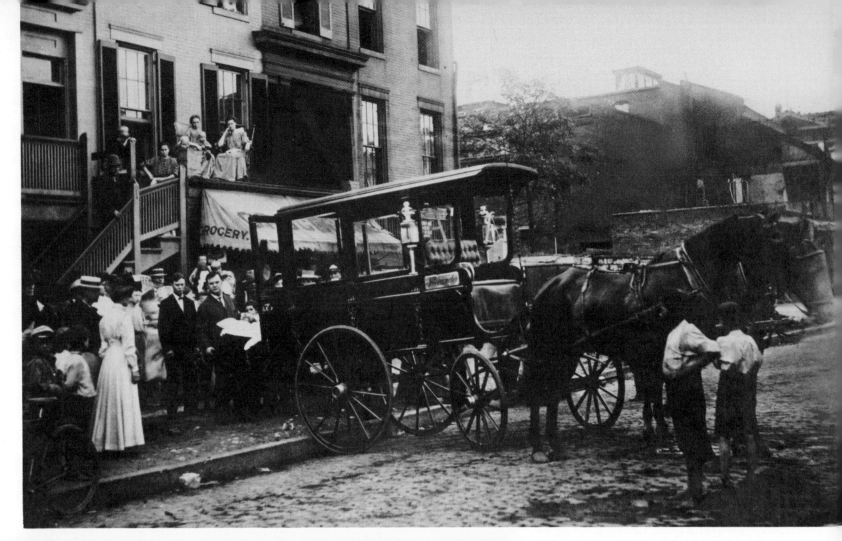

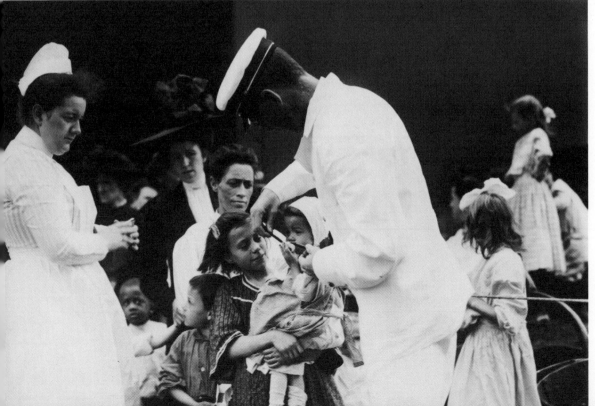

Above: Victim of Tuberculosis. Photograph, c. 1908. [M.H.S.] This Minnesota patient is being taken to the hospital by ambulance. *Left* and *below:* Floating Hospital. Photographs, c. 1910. [L.C.] Boats were occasionally used as tuberculosis camps to isolate the diseased and provide them with fresh air.

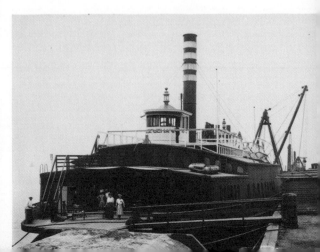

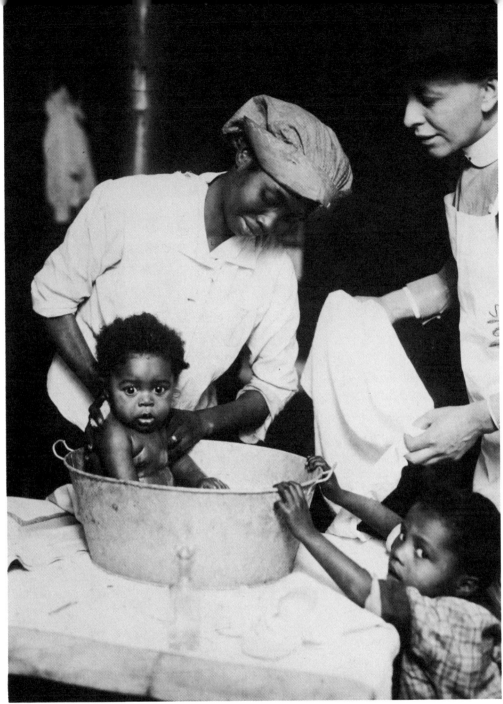

Left: Infant Welfare Society Nurse. Photograph, c. 1907. [C.H.S.] The Infant Welfare Society sponsored a visiting nurse program to care for slum children. Here a nurse teaches a mother how best to bathe her baby. *Below left:* Visiting Nurse in a Settlement House. Photograph, early 1900s. [V.N.S.N.Y.] *Below right:* Preparing Daily Supply of Dressings. Photograph, c. 1900. [N.M.H.T.] Bandages were handmade by the nursing staff of New York's German Dispensary, now Lenox Hill Hospital.

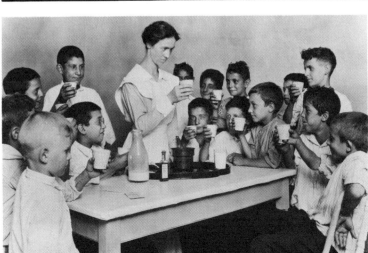

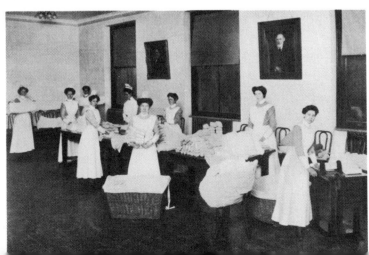

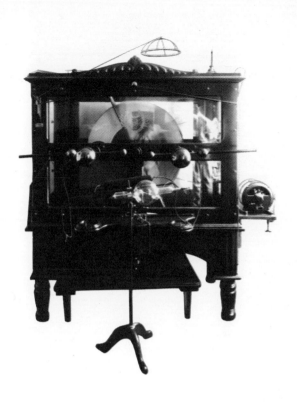

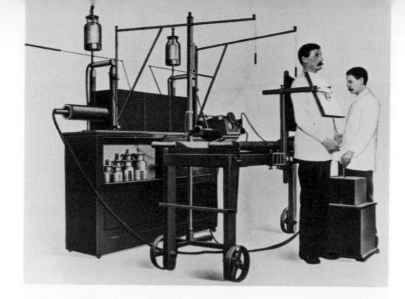

Left: Static Electric Machine with X-Ray Apparatus. Photograph, c. 1880–1900. [N.M.H.T.] Initially the electric motor on the right was used to start circular glass plates inside the machine which in turn produced static electricity. *Above:* An Early 20th Century X-Ray Machine. Photograph, early 1900s. [N.M.H.T.] This illustration appeared in the book *Notes on X-light* by William Rollins.

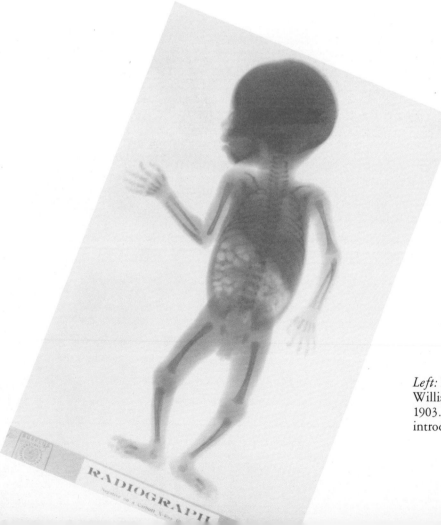

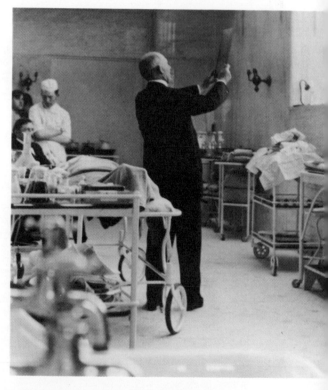

Left: X-Ray of Baby Boy. Photograph, c. 1900. [N.M.H.T.] *Above:* William Stewart Halsted Examining an X-Ray Plate. Photograph, c. 1903. [N.L.M.] The noted Professor of Surgery at Johns Hopkins introduced the use of rubber gloves in surgery.

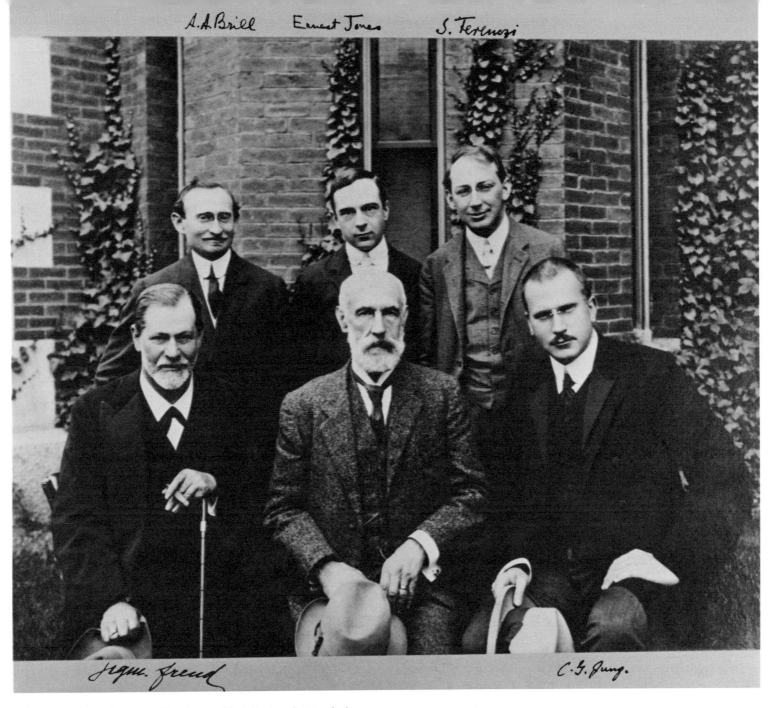

A.A.Brill   Ernest Jones   S. Ferenczi

Sigm. Freud   C.G. Jung.

Above: Psychoanalysts Participating at Clark University Psychology Conference, 1909. Photograph. [M.23.] At the invitation of Clark's President, Granville Stanley Hall (front row center), the celebrated European psychoanalysts C.G. Jung (front row, right) and Sigmund Freud (front row, left) visited America, where Freud delivered his first lectures in this country at Clark. *Right:* Treatment Room at the Adams Nervine Asylum, Boston. Photograph, c. 1904. [N.L.M.] At the turn of the century, treatment for sufferers from hysteria included electrotherapy and hot baths. Shown here is the electric room.

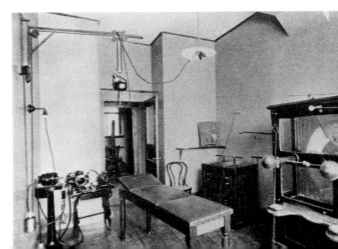

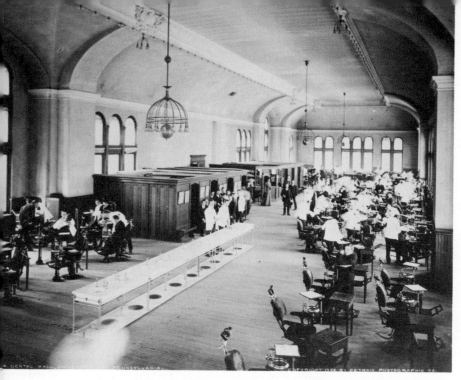

Above: Dental Hall, University of Pennsylvania. Photograph, c. 1904. [L.C.] The University of Pennsylvania was an early and prominent center for the study of dentistry, as it was for medical education. *Above right:* Dr. Olga A. Lentz. Photograph, c. 1910. [M.H.S.] Dr. Lentz practiced in St. Paul, Minnesota, in the early 1900s. *Below right:* Dental Class at the University of Minnesota. Photograph, c. 1900. [M.H.S.]

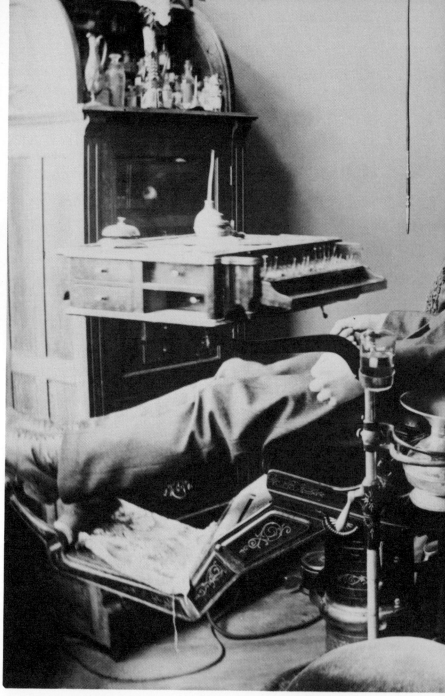

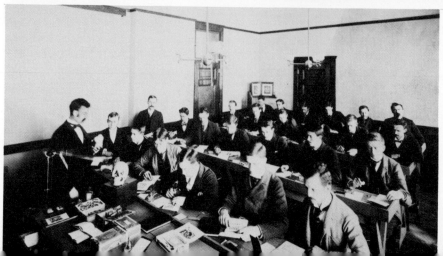

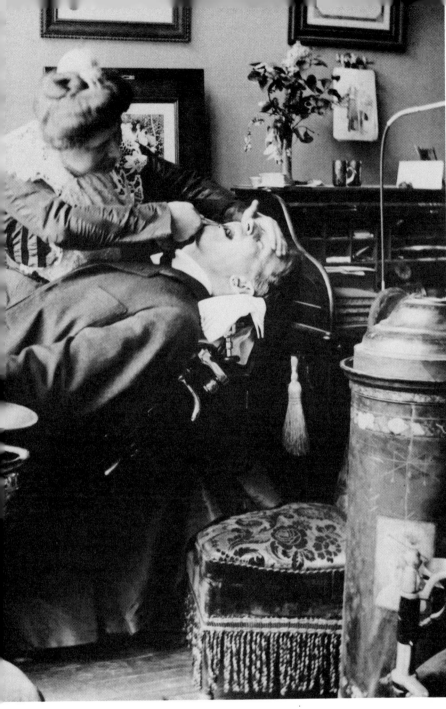

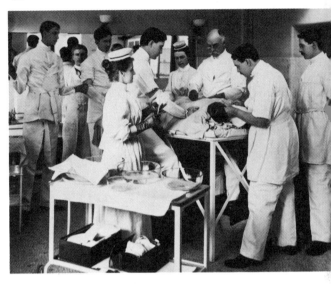

Below: Professor Charles McBurney Operating in Roosevelt Hospital, New York. Photograph, early 20th century. [N.L.M.] He was known for locating the point of pain —"McBurney's Point"—which indicated appendicitis.

Below left: Operating Room, Freeman's Hospital. Photograph, c. 1908. [M.24.] The Freeman's Hospital Clinic was a black medical center in Washington, D.C. *Below:* Drs. C.H. and W.J. Mayo. Photograph, 1905. [M.H.S.] In the early years of the century, just as today, institutions were deemed outstanding when those who practiced in them were outstanding. In Rochester, Minnesota, the Mayo Clinic gained worldwide fame under the leadership of Charles and William Mayo.

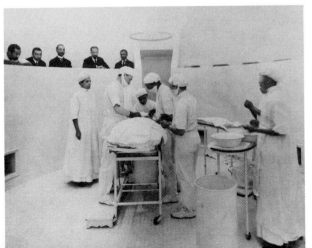

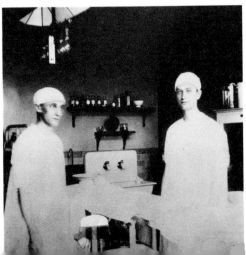

113

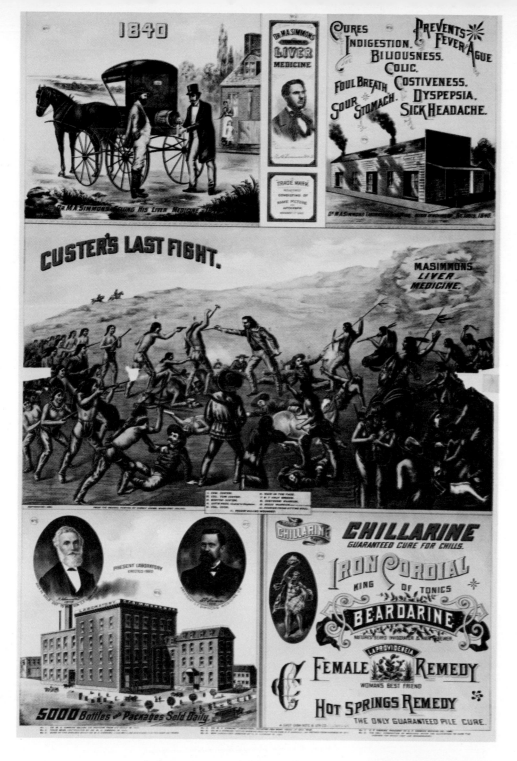

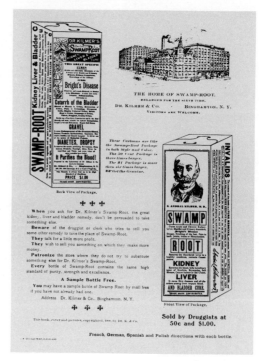

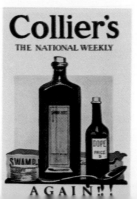

Left: Custer's Last Fight. Advertising poster, late 19th century. [L.C.] In addition to the view of Custer at Little Big Horn, this poster traces the rise of Dr. M.A. Simmon's fortune. In 1842 he founded a "modest" laboratory in Mississippi; by 1883 the firm was well-established in St. Louis; by the end of the century it claimed daily sales of 5,000 packages of patent medicines. *Above:* Swamp-Root Advertisement. Print, c. 1900. [S.H.S.W.] Its advice to the consumer: "Beware of the druggist or clerk who tries to sell you some other remedy to take the place of Swamp-Root." *Below: Collier's* Magazine Cover. Print, 1912. [P.C.] The fakery of patent medicine advertising was exposed by Samuel Hopkins Adams in a remarkable series of articles appearing in *Collier's* in 1905-06. Stirred by the articles, the medical and pharmaceutical professions, and responsible drug manufacturers, lobbied for the landmark Pure Food and Drug Act, which Congress passed in 1906.

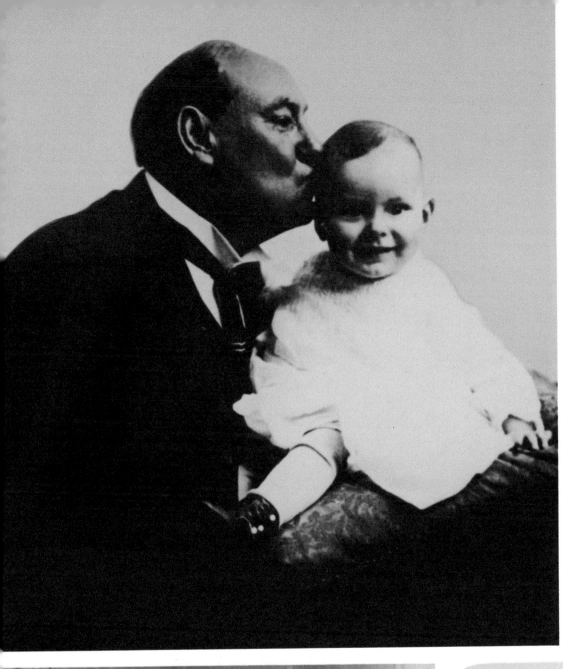

Left: Dr. Harvey Washington Wiley. Photograph, early 20th century. [A.P.A.] Dr. Wiley, a leading proponent of the Pure Food and Drug Act, is seen demonstrating "Osculatio Antiseptica" (antiseptic kissing), which failed to catch on. *Below left:* Mead Johnson & Co. Booth at American Medical Association Convention. Photograph, early 20th century. [M.J.C.] Reputable drug houses and the professional associations lent support to the government's reforms. *Below right:* The United States Pharmacopoeia Members. Photograph, 1900. [A.P.A.] Members of the group, which periodically sets standards for drugs, pose in Mt. Vernon, Virginia, in 1900.

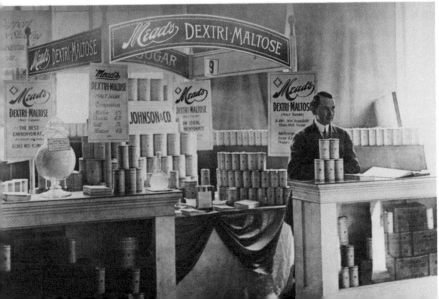

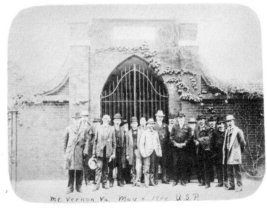

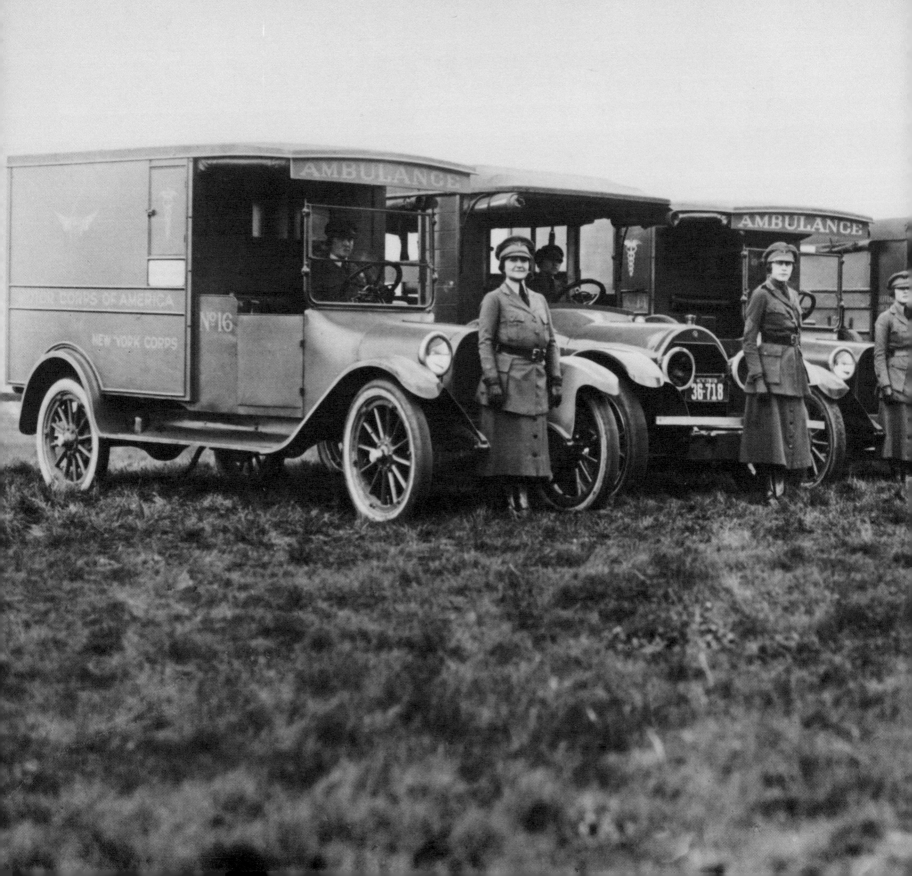

CHAPTER SEVEN

1910-1919

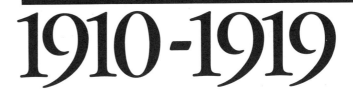

On May 5, 1915, Dr. Ludwig Kast addressed the Roentgen Ray Society of New York City. The occasion was the twentieth anniversary of Professor Wilhelm Conrad Roentgen's universally acclaimed discovery of the x-ray: "To look through the living chest; to see the shadows of the heart, the expansion of the lung and the heaving of the diaphragm was a thrilling experience and full of suggestion. The discovery carried the eye . . . into the human tissues . . .

"Both in surgery and internal medicine the practical value of the method was quickly appreciated, and never perhaps has a method of examination been introduced into medicine and surgery which so promptly and so universally won acceptance and appreciation as did radiology. It made possible better therapeutic results; it curtailed suffering; it saved human lives."

Roentgen's work may have been in Germany, but the impact of the x-ray on surgery and medical and biological research in the United States was revolutionary. Following World War I, when the army trained radiologists to treat the wounded, growing numbers of physicians recognized the unique value of the x-ray in medical diagnosis and therapy.

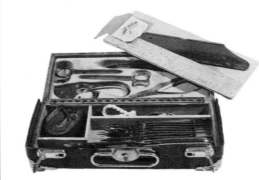

Technical advances occurred rapidly in all fields of medicine in the first three decades of this century and the number of new instruments and techniques invented was vast. In short, medicine was becoming the sophisticated and complex science it is today.

Left: Ambulance Corps in World War I. Photograph, 1917. [F.L.I.] *Above:* World War I U.S. Army Surgical Kit. Mixed materials, 1917. [H.M.S.]

1910: 91,972,266 inhabitants; 45.7% urban, 54.3% rural
Mann Act declared white slavery illegal

1911: First transcontinental plane flight; 84 hours, 2 minutes

1912: Woodrow Wilson elected President
New Mexico, Arizona became 47th, 48th states
1912-25: U.S. intervention in Nicaragua

1913: 16th and 17th Amendments adopted
Federal Reserve system authorized

1914: Clayton Antitrust Act
July-August: War began in Europe
U.S. proclaimed neutrality in WW I

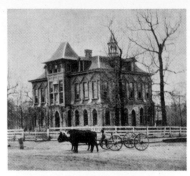

Many Rural Medical Colleges Closed

1910: The course of medical education was changed by Abraham Flexner's (1866-1959), report on Canadian medical schools, *Medical Education in the United States and Canada*. It hastened needed reforms in the organization of the medical schools.

1910: A course in public health nursing was established at Columbia University.

1911: A spine fusion operation, devised by New York orthopedist Russell Hibbs, revolutionized the treatment of spinal tuberculosis and scoliosis.

1911: Dietary experiments by a Polish-born biochemist, Casimir Funk, led to the discovery and naming of vitamins. Funk, who suggested the existence of vitamins B_1, B_2, C, and D, emigrated to the United States in 1915.

1911: The first American-designed electrocardiograph was installed at Rockefeller Hospital. It was so well made that it was used for the next 32 years.

1912: Vitamin A was discovered by Thomas B. Osborne (1859-1929), and Lafayette B. Mendel (1872-1935), at Yale; and Elmer V. McCollum (1879-1967), at the University of Wisconsin.

1912: Phenobarbital, a crystalline compound used as an important sedative, was introduced.

1912: The U.S. Public Health Service adopted its present name. Even though the federal government's emphasis switched to public health, the Service continued to care for sick and disabled sailors, its original function.

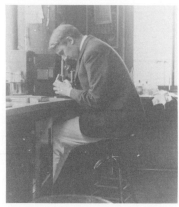

Graduate Student at Johns Hopkins

1912: Coronary thrombosis, which had gone unrecognized in the United States for years, was given its first classic description in English, by James B. Herrick (1861-1954), professor of medicine at Rush Medical College, Chicago. Herrick's famous paper, "Clinical Features of Sudden Obstruction of the Coronary Arteries," was published in the *Journal of the A.M.A.*

1912: Tissue culture, the growth of living cells in an artificial medium, was achieved in 1907 by Ross G. Harrison (1870-1954), at Johns Hopkins. Public attention was caught by the amazing fact that animal cells could be grown in flasks and were capable of outliving the body from which they had been taken. On January 17, 1912, surgeon Alexis Carrel started a culture of cells from the heart of an embryonic chick. Regularly transplanted to a fresh medium, the heart culture continued to grow until 1946—two years after the surgeon's death and 34 years after the cells had been removed from the chick.

1913: John J. Abel and his associates at Johns Hopkins first isolated amino acids from the blood while studying proteins.

1913: Full-time clinical professorships were initiated at Johns Hopkins. For the first time, clinical teachers no longer had to augment part-time salaries with fees from private practice.

1913: The first artificial kidney was developed. A mechanical system which freed a dog's blood of toxic chemicals by circulating it through collodion tubing was developed by John Jacob Abel, L.G. Rowntree and B.B. Turner. Toxins passed out of the tubing into surrounding liquid, leaving the blood inside. The technique of vividiffusion, or hemodialysis as we know it today, was not used on humans until the 1940s, when more efficient tubing and safe anticoagulants had been developed.

1913: The Rockefeller Foundation established by John D. Rockefeller, Sr., began a world-wide program for the study and control of hookworm, malaria and yellow fever. During its first 14 years, the Foundation was given $183 million by Rockefeller.

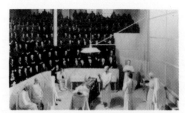

Dr. John B. Murphy's Surgical Clinic at Mercy Hospital, Chicago

1913: The American College of Surgeons was founded. The national organization sponsored an annual two-week congress of operative clinics, thus marking professional recognition that the practice of surgery required special training.

1915: U.S. Coast Guard established
Federal Trade Commission created

1916: Wilson reelected President
U.S. troops entered Mexico
Federal 8-hour work day law passed
1916-39: Louis Brandeis, Justice of
Supreme Court

1917: Puerto Ricans given U.S. citizenship
April: Declaration of War
Selective Service inaugurated

1918: Wilson stated war aims in Fourteen Points
Creation of National War Labor Board
November 11: Armistice

1919: Wilson won Nobel Peace Prize
18th Amendment (Prohibition) ratified

1919

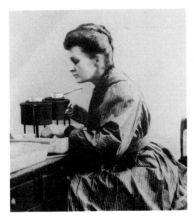

Dr. Marie Curie

1913: Radium, discovered in 1898 by Pierre and Marie Curie in France, was discovered to have a palliative effect on malignant tumors.

1914: Pasteurization of milk began in major cities.

1914: The first list of hospitals approved for intern training was published by the A.M.A. It numbered 508 general hospitals, with openings for 2,667 interns. An additional 60 special hospitals and 35 state institutions for the insane offered another 428 internships.

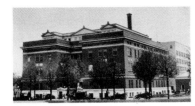

Mayo Clinic

1914: New building of the Mayo Clinic opened in Rochester. The following year the Mayo brothers and their partners incorporated the Mayo Foundation for Medical Education and Research

1915: Death certificates came into general use.

1915: Pellagra, widespread in the Southern states, was found to be caused by a dietary deficiency, not by infection as previously believed. The discoverer was Joseph Golberger, a U.S. Public Health physician. The pellagra-preventive factor, isolated in 1926, was named Vitamin G in his honor.

1915: Women doctors were admitted to full membership in the American Medical Association. In this same year the Medical Women's National Association was formed.

1915: The American College of Physicians incorporated and held its first meeting in New York City. Headquarters were moved from New York to Chicago in 1921; by 1925, when it moved again to Philadelphia, the ACP counted some 1,000 members.

1915: The thyroid hormone, named thyroxin, was isolated and chemically identified by biochemist Edward C. Kendall at the Mayo Clinic.

1915: The Catholic Hospital Association was formed.

1916: Heparin, a complex organic acid capable of preventing blood clotting under certain circumstances, was discovered by Jay McLean and William H. Howell at Johns Hopkins. In 1929 heparin was first used experimentally to prevent venous thrombosis.

1916: The Johns Hopkins School of Hygiene and Public Health was founded. It opened in Baltimore in 1918.

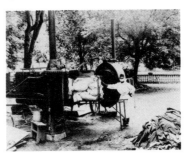

American Red Cross Sterilizer in France

1917: After the U.S. entry into World War I, army training camps brought together city boys carrying urban contagious diseases and country boys, who had not been exposed to them and therefore lacked immunity. The result was thousands of cases of measles, mumps, cerebrospinal meningitis, influenza and pneumonia. During the war, 53,000 soliders and sailors were killed in action or died from wounds. They were outnumbered by the 63,000 who died from disease.

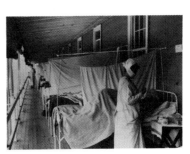

Influenza Ward, Walter Reed Army Hospital

1918: A global epidemic of influenza killed nearly half a million Americans, caused 21 million deaths worldwide. The serious form of the epidemic reached the U.S. in October. Emergency hospitals were set up in churches, schools and public buildings. The epidemic lasted until 1919, and the rates of illness and death were so high that the nation's economy suffered.

1919: At the end of World War I, sympathy for mutilated veterans gave rise to the concept of rehabilitation. Training schools, hospitals and special institutes were founded.

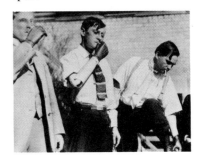

World War I Veterans with Artifical Limbs

Right: Making Rounds. Photograph, 1915. [U.S.A.] Doctors, nurses and medical students tour the wards of Mobile City Hospital. *Below:* Dr. Joseph Smith. Photograph, 1913. [S.H.S.W.] Dr. Smith practiced in Wausau, Wisconsin. He is seen posed next to his Model T Ford. *Below right:* Bringing in a Patient. Photograph, early 20th century. [U.S.A.] The Emerald-Hodgson Hospital of Sewanee. Tennessee served the University of the South, and the area's mountain people.

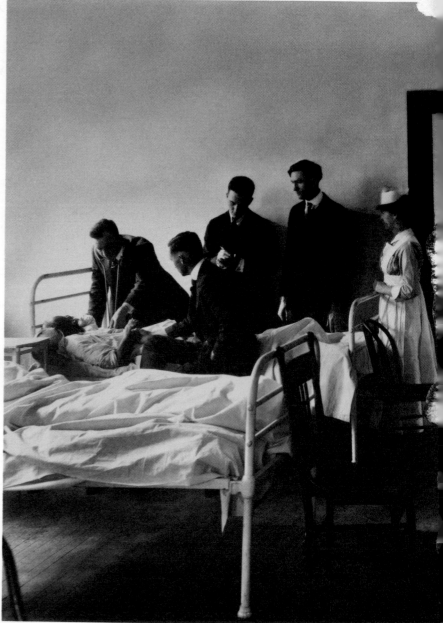

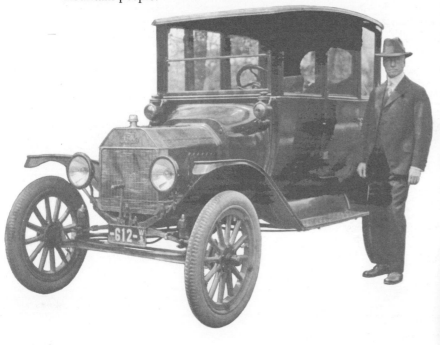

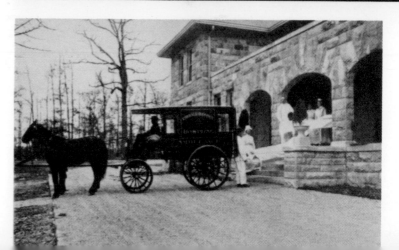

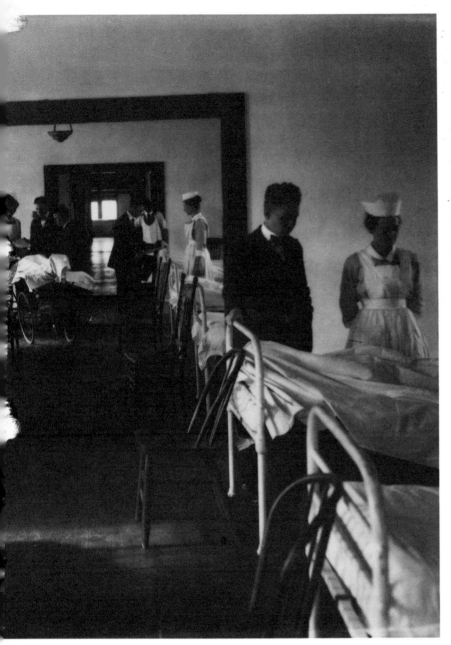

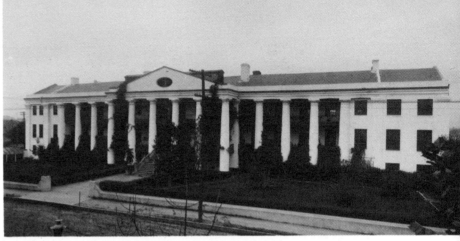

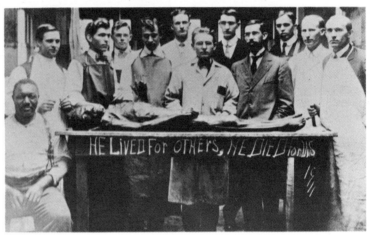

Top: Mobile City Hospital. Photograph, c. 1910. [U.S.A.] *Above:* Medical Students. Photograph, 1911. [A.H.S.] An Atlanta Medical College dissection class chalked on their table: ''He lived for others, he died for us.'' *Below:* Mobile Medical College. Photograph, c. 1913. [U.S.A.] In a view taken by Mobile photographer Erik Overbey (glass plate negative broken), medical students are seen at work in the dissecting room.

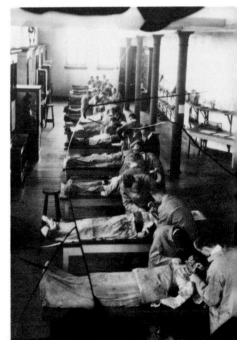

Dept. of Public Health, Div. of Sanitation F. No. 6

DIPHTHERIA

KEEP OUT OF THIS HOUSE

By Order ot BOARD OF HEALTH

HEALTH OFFICER

Any person removing this card without authority is liable to prosecution

Above: Quarantine Poster. Print, c. 1915. [N.L.M.] Despite advances in the prevention and treatment of diseases, all too frequently epidemics broke out across the country. This diphtheria poster was used in San Francisco.

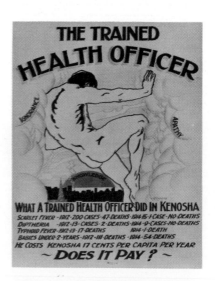

Above: Public Health Poster. Print, 1915. [S.H.S.W.] In Kenosha, Wisconsin, the city government advertised for support of its public health program. *Right:* Examination of Rats Suspected of Carrying Bubonic Plague. Photograph, 1914. [N.L.M.]

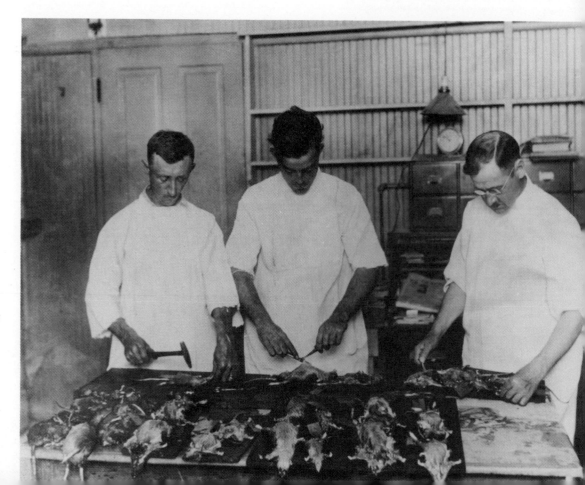

Krusen Stops All Sales and Deliveries by Liquor Dealers

City Health Board Prohibits All Sale or Delivery of Liquor

SOUTH PHILADELPHIA SECTION CLEANED BY VARE SHOWS HEAVIEST MORTALITY RATE IN THE CITY

Fourth of Whole Number in Area Where He Holds Contracts

RESIDENTS, DESPERATE, WILL APPEAL TO COURT

Eminent Italian Artist Enters Lists in Behalf of Countrymen

More than one-fourth of the 2234 deaths which occurred in Philadelphia for the week ending at noon yesterday were in the Third street-cleaning district, or that section of the city south of South street, between the Delaware and Schuylkill Rivers, for which State Senator Edwin H. Vare holds the contract.

Of the unprecedented toll of deaths, more than 80 per cent were due to epidemic influenza and resulting pneumonia, the wide and rapid spread of which, a score or more of the city's most prominent physicians and authorities on public health and sanitation have unqualifiedly declared, was largely due to the atmospheric circulation, the germ-laden dirt and filth that remained in the public highways. Particularly, said the foremost of them, did that condition prevail in the sections where Senator Vare held the lucrative contracts.

Eight hundred and eighteen deaths in the nine wards below South street in one week have drawn the deadly parallel between the disinterested statements of medical authorities and the denial of dirty streets by Senator Vare and the attempted backing up of that denial by Chief Hicks, of the Street Cleaning Bureau, whose son in public opinion was a fine upon Vare of $645, a penalty so trivial as to cause a laugh throughout City Hall, where real conditions are known.

It required the authority and the action of Director Krusen, of the Department of Public Health and Charities, to force a clean-up of the streets by flushing, and the rather enfoumatical statement made then by Senator Vare, that the streets were no dirtier than they always had been, stands in further contrast, in view of the indictment brought by disinterested medical authorities, with the fact that the largest number of deaths in any one ward in the city occurred in the Thirty-ninth, where Senator Vare

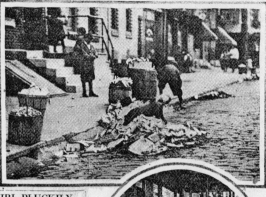

GIRL PLUCKILY ROUTS WRECKER GANG ON P. R. R.

Uniontown Operator Sets Signal as Bullets Graze Body

Special Telegram to Public Ledger

Uniontown, Pa., Oct. 12.—Barricading herself in the "HY" tower of the Pennsylvania Railroad at Gist passing, near here, after she had discovered and fired upon would-be train wreckers, Miss E. M. Vensel, tower operator, pluckily held her post. Despite a heavy revolver attack, she kept the gang at bay until the arrival of a freight train, the crew of which put the attackers to rout.

The young woman's pluck prevented the wrecking of at least one

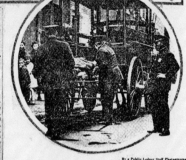

The upper picture shows one of the streets in South Philadelphia where

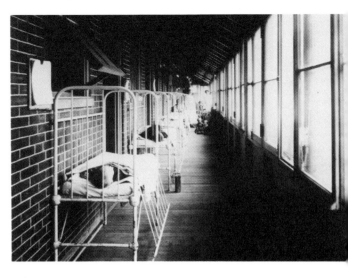

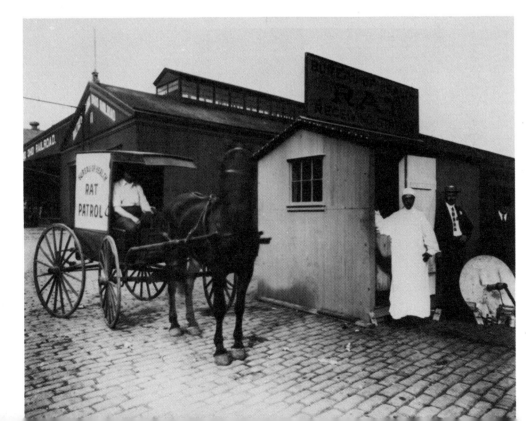

Above: Whooping Cough Ward. Photograph, c. 1910. [N.L.M.] Fresh air was part of the prescribed treatment for whooping cough at Philadelphia General Hospital. *Above left:* News of Influenza Epidemic. Newspaper clippings, 1918. [P.C.] In 1793 Philadelphia was struck by a yellow fever epidemic, in 1832 with cholera, and in 1918 influenza ravaged the city, felling as many as 4,000 people in a day. With neither vaccine nor medicine, one leading physician prescribed staying home and drinking as much whiskey as possible. *Below left:* Rat Patrol. Photograph, early 20th century. [N.L.M.] Philadelphia's Bureau of Health waged a campaign against the disease-carrying rodents.

The series of discoveries which, in its application to surgery, has brought about the present antiseptic and aseptic methods of operation, is concerned both with the shape or use of the instruments of surgery and with their preparation for use. The mere sterilization, by boiling or by steaming, of all instruments and dressings, is enough to ensure their freedom from the ordinary micro-organisms of suppuration; but the surgeon cannot boil or steam either himself or his patient. The preparation, therefore, of the surgeon's hands, and of the skin over the area of operation, is made not only by scrubbing with soap and hot water, but by careful use of antiseptic lotions. Again, ligatures and sutures, which must be kept in stock ready for use, are kept, after careful sterilization, in antiseptic lotion, or are again sterilized immediately before an operation. Again, all towels used at an operation must be prepared, either by sterilization or by immersion in antiseptic lotion.

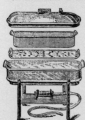

FIG. 13—Instrument Sterilizer.

The sterilization of all instruments and dressings is a simple matter: the usual sterilizer is a vessel like a fish-kettle, with a perforated metal tray in it, so that the instruments can be immersed in boiling water, and can be lifted on the tray and transferred straight from the sterilizer into vessels containing sterilized water or antiseptic lotion. For the sterilization of dressings an upper vessel is fitted to the sterilizer, so that the steam may permeate the dressings placed in it. In hospital practice it is used also to sterilize all towels, aprons and the like in a large cylindrical vessel. Sterilization by boiling or steaming, together with the use of antiseptic lotions, or of water that has been boiled, for all such things as cannot be boiled or steamed, is the essential principle of the surgery of the present day; and practically the antiseptic method and the aseptic method have become one, varying a little this way or that according to the nature and circumstances of the case.

Beside anaesthetics and antiseptics, there is a third series of discoveries that has profoundly influenced surgery—the use of the forces of electricity. The uses of electricity are fivefold.
1. *The Galvano-Cautery.*—The original form of the cautery, the *fer ardent* of Paré's time, for the arrest of haemorrhage after amputation, was a terrible affair. Happily for mankind, his invention of the ligature put an end to this use of the cautery, but it was still used in a small number of other cases. Subsequently Claude André Paquelin (b. 1836) invented a very ingenious form of cautery, a series of metal blades or points of different shapes and sizes, that could be fitted to a handle: these points were hollow inside, and were filled with fine platinum gauze, and, by means of a bottle and hand-bellows, they could be kept heated with benzene-vapour. Thus, when they had once been raised to a glowing heat by holding them

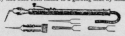

FIG. 14.—Galvano-cautery Set.

over a spirit-lamp, they could be kept at any desired heat. This instrument is still in use for a few cases where very rapid and extensive cauterization is necessary. But for all finer use of actual heat the galvano-cautery alone is used—a series of very minute points of platinum, with a suitable trigger-handle, connected with a battery or (by means of a converter) with the ordinary house supply of electricity. In this way it is possible to apply a glowing point with a fineness and accuracy of adjustment that were wholly impossible with Paquelin's cautery.
2. *Electrolysis.*—This method is of great value, in suitable cases, for the arrest or obliteration of small growths. The passage of the electric current between needles introduced into or under the skin brings about a gradual shrinking or cicatrization of the tissues subjected to it, without the production of any unsightly scar.

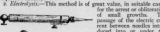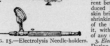

FIG. 15.—Electrolysis Needle-holders.
3. *Electro-Motor Power.*—During recent years the use of a small electro-motor machine has come into the practice of surgery for certain operations on the bones; especially for the operation for disease involving the mastoid bone. It is, of course, a better method for the use of a fine drill or burr, for example, than the "dental engine," where the power is generated by a pedal turning a wheel, and it will probably come into wide use both for dental surgery and for those operations of general surgery that require very gradual and delicate removal of small circumscribed areas of bone, especially of the cranial bones.
4. *The X-Rays.*—This, the most unexpected and, as it were, the most sensational discovery that has been bestowed on physicians and surgeons since the discovery of anaesthetics, is now used over a very wide and varied field of practice. Its value does not stop at the detection and localization of foreign bodies; indeed, this is but a small part of its work. It is used constantly for cases of actual or suspected fracture or dislocation; for cases of congenital or acquired

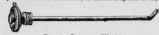

FIG. 16.—Cystoscope (Nitze's).

deformity; for cases involving difficulties of diagnosis between a swelling of the bone due to inflammation and a swelling due to a tumour; and for obscure cases of spinal disease, hip disease and the like. Moreover, it has been found possible, by Dr Hugh Walsham, and others to obtain pictures of the thoracic organs that are a very valuable guide in many obscure cases of disease of the lungs or of the pleura, and in many cases of thoracic aneurism or of intra-thoracic tumour. Every year the number and the range of the cases where the X-rays are helpful for diagnosis and for treatment become greater; and it is impossible to say at what point the surgical value of this discovery will find its limits. Beyond these uses, it is probable that the X-rays will find and extend the importance that they already have in the direct treatment of certain cases of disease of the skin (see X-RAY TREATMENT).
5. *The Electric Light.*—Beside the general superiority of this light to other lights for the routine work of surgery, there are several special uses for it. Of these, the most important is the *cystoscope,* a long narrow tube, shaped and curved somewhat like a catheter, and having at its end a very minute glow-lamp and reflector, and a small window. Its other end is fitted with a lens, and is connected by a switch with the main current. With this instrument, in skilled hands, it is possible to inspect the interior of the bladder, and in many cases to make an exact diagnosis under circumstances where otherwise it would be impossible. Another instance of the value of the electric lamp in diagnosis is given by the trans-illumination of the facial bones in cases of suspected disease of the central cavity of the superior maxillary bone. A small glow-lamp is held in the closed mouth, in a darkened room, and by a comparison of the shadows on the two sides of the face, thus trans-illuminated, an exact diagnosis can often be obtained as to the presence or absence of pus in this central cavity. Again, a small glow-lamp, duly sterilized, is often of great value in deep operations on the abdominal cavity.
The bactericidal properties of light have long been demonstrated by Bie and others. Professor Niels Finsen of Copenhagen first used the ultra-violet rays of solar light in the treatment of skin diseases.

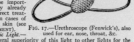

FIG. 17.—Urethroscope (Fenwick's), also used for ear, nose, throat, &c.

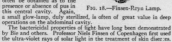

FIG. 18.—Finsen-Reyn Lamp.

Above: Surgical Instruments and Appliances. Book page, 1911. [N.Y.P. L./P.C.] The technology of medical instruments and devices made major advances in the early 1900s. Here, a page from a book published in 1911 describing such "discoveries."

Below: Otoscope. 1913. Metal. [N.M.H.T.] This battery-lighted device, with a lens, enabled physicians to examine the inside of the ear. *Bottom:* Mastoid Cases. Photograph, 1912. [C.H.S.] Before the discovery of penicillin, infection of the ear required mastoid surgery. This portrait of post-operative patients was taken in the children's ward of Cook County Contagious Hospital in Chicago.

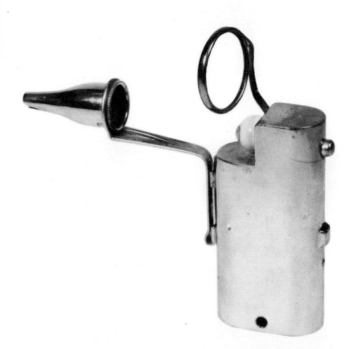

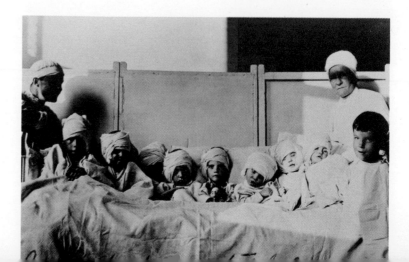

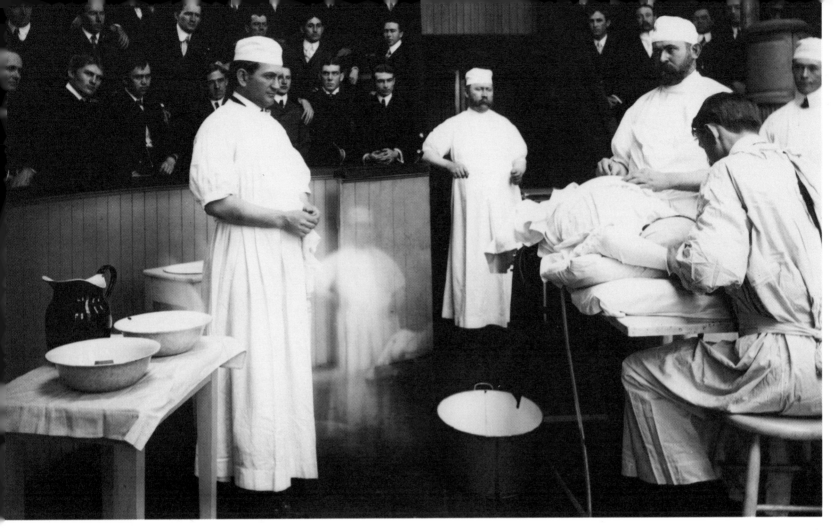

Above: Mobile City Hospital Operating Theater. Photograph, early 20th century. [H.M.P.S.] Drs. Howard, Frazer and Jackson are demonstrating an operation. *Below left:* John J. Abel. Photograph, early 20th century. [M.14.] In 1913, Dr. Abel of Johns Hopkins and two colleagues published their design for the first artificial kidney device. The process, then termed ''vividiffusion,'' is known today as hemodialysis. *Below right:* Vividiffusion Device. Mixed materials, c. 1913. [M.12.] The original artificial kidney, and Abel's notes describing its design.

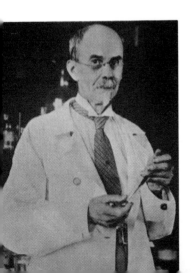

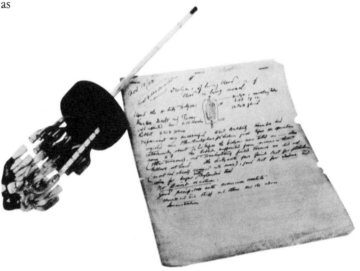

125

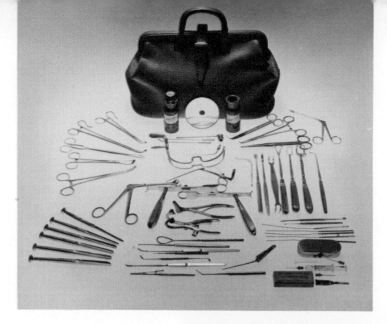

Left: Physician's Bag and Contents. Mixed materials, early 20th century. [H.M.S.] The Historical Museum of Medicine and Dentistry of the Hartford Medical Society exhibits the instruments of Dr. George F. Vail who, beginning in 1910, limited his practice to the speciality of Eye, Ear, Nose and Throat. *Below:* Restored Country Doctor's Office. Photograph, 20th century. [P.C.P.S.] The Mütter Medical Museum of Philadelphia's College of Physicians and Surgeons has installed a typical country doctor's office of the early 1900s. Like numbers of his colleagues, Dr. Philip Gordon Kitchen, who practiced here, did not have running water, as the washstand and pitcher in the background attest.

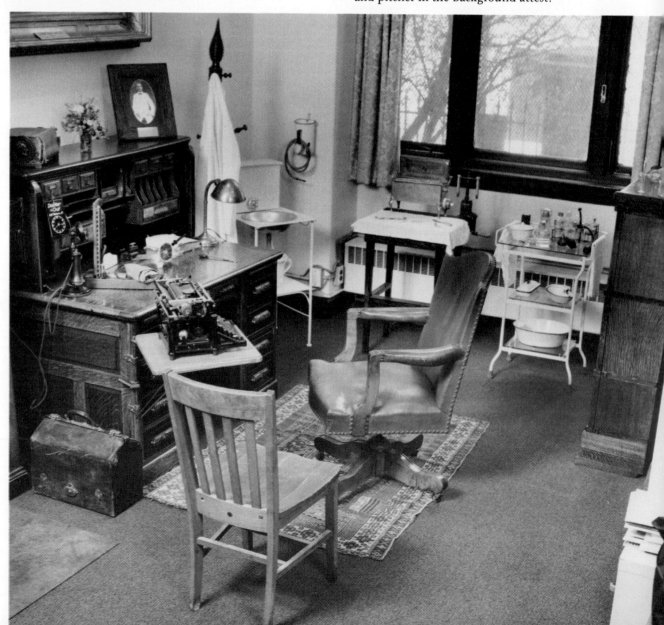

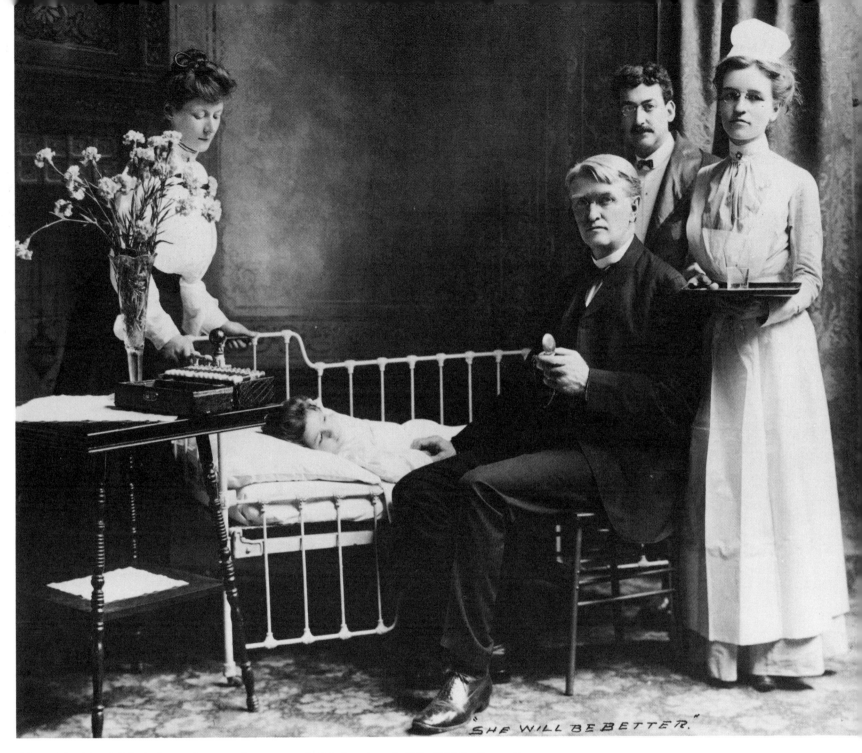

"SHE WILL BE BETTER."

Above: Physician With Patient. Photograph, c. 1900. [L.C.] Captioned, "She Will Be Better," this picture was carefully posed by a Chicago photographer, possibly W.H. Willard Jones.

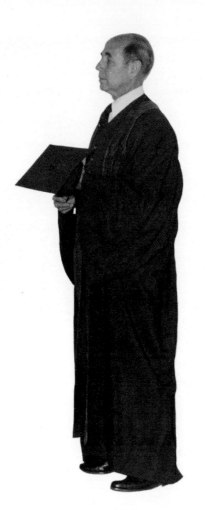

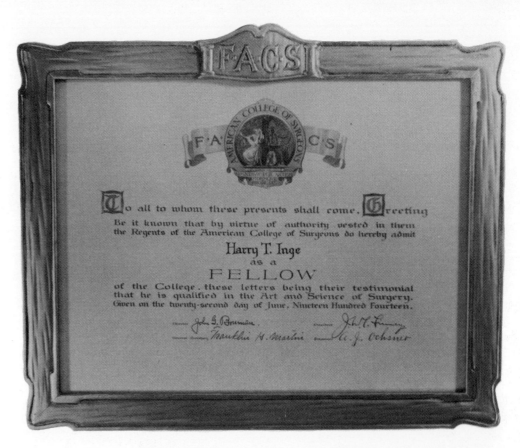

Left: Cap and Gown. Fabric, c. 1914. [H.M.M.] *Above:* Certificate, 1914. [H.M.M.] Dr. Harry T. Inge of Mobile, Alabama was named a Fellow of the American College of Surgeons in 1914. The cap and gown, modeled here by Dr. Samuel Eichold, Curator of Mobile's Heustis Medical Museum, were worn at the College on ceremonial occasions. *Below:* The Pasteur-Lister Gavel of the Society of Clinical Surgery. Mixed materials, early 20th century. [P.C.P.S.] This gavel is made of a doorknob from Pasteur's home and the leg of Lister's dressing table in the Glasgow Infirmary.

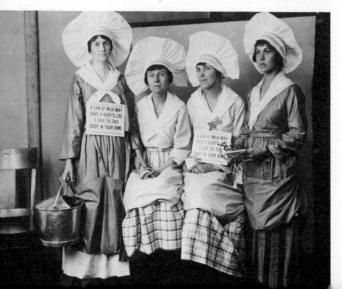

Left: "Milk Ladies." Photograph, 1917. [C.H.S.] Society ladies in Chicago dressed as milk maids to raise money for children in settlement houses.

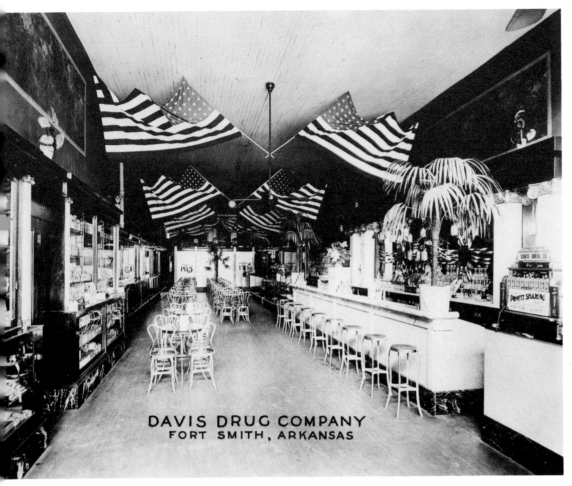

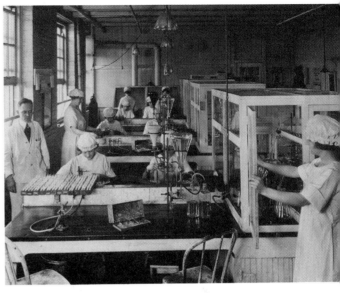

Left: The Davis Drugstore. Photograph, early 20th century. [L.C.] *Above:* Ampoule Filling Department, Eli Lilly and Company. Photograph, c. 1917. [E.L.C.] *Below left:* Norwich Pharmacal Company Analytical Laboratory. Photograph, early 20th century. [M.25.] Dr. M.W. Stofer, Norwich's medical director, is on the left; H.J. Broughton, probably a chemist, is on the right. *Below right:* Dress Uniform of the U.S. Public Health Service. 1914. [N.L.M.]

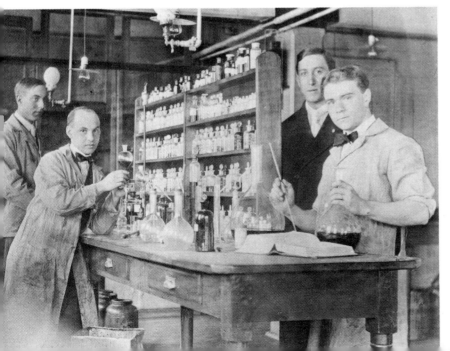

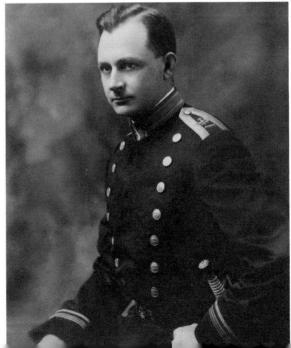

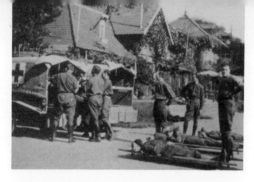

Above: Evacuating Wounded in France. Photogaph, 1918. [J.J.] World War I U.S. Army Medical Corpsmen are shown at a field aid station loading wounded for transport to hospitals at the rear. *Right:* Ambulance Airplane. Photograph, 1918. [N.L.M.] A DeHavilland biplane, adapted for transporting the wounded, is shown in flight over Langley Field, Virginia. *Below:* Red Cross Volunteers Providing Refreshments for Soldiers Aboard a Troop Train. Photograph c. 1918. [L.C.]

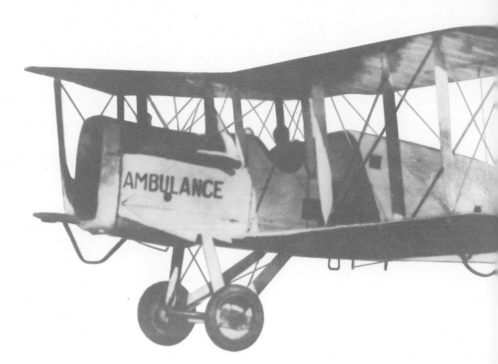

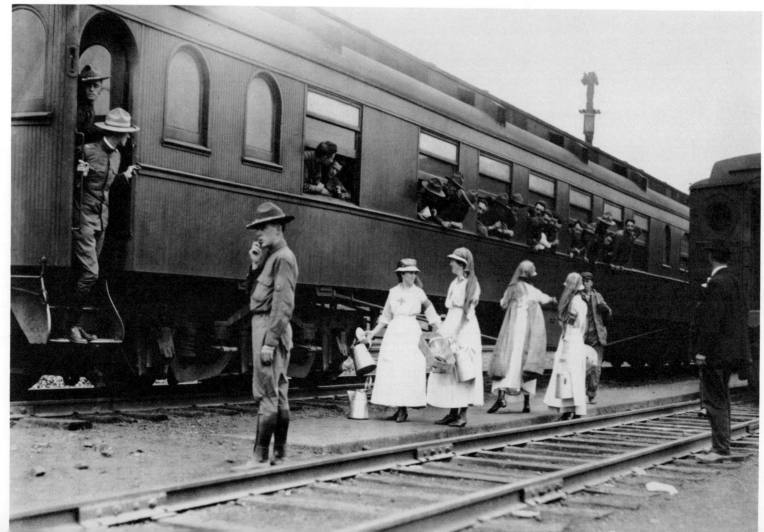

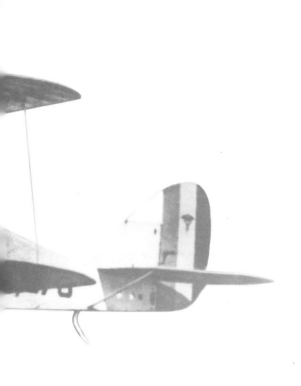

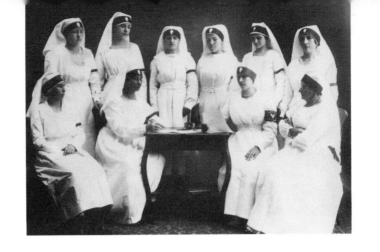

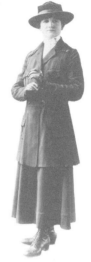

Above: Polish-American Volunteer Nurses. Photograph, c. 1918. [M.26.] This group, under the auspices of the Polish National Aid Committee, was only one of many groups of patriotic volunteers. *Right top to bottom:* Nurses' Uniforms, World War I. Photographs, c. 1918. [L.C.] Three styles worn by Red Cross nurses. *Left:* Operating Team, U.S. Marine Hospital, Staten Island, New York. Photograph, 1919. [N.L.M.] The identifiable are: Dr. Heart, Chief of Surgery, Miss Samuelson, Anesthetist (seen dripping anesthetic on a gauze mask over the patient's face), and Dr. Patty Graciano, Assistant.

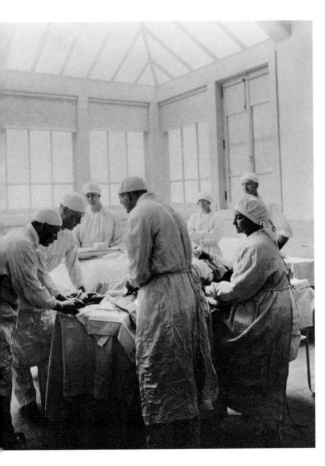

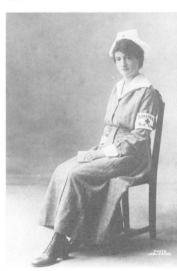

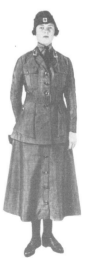

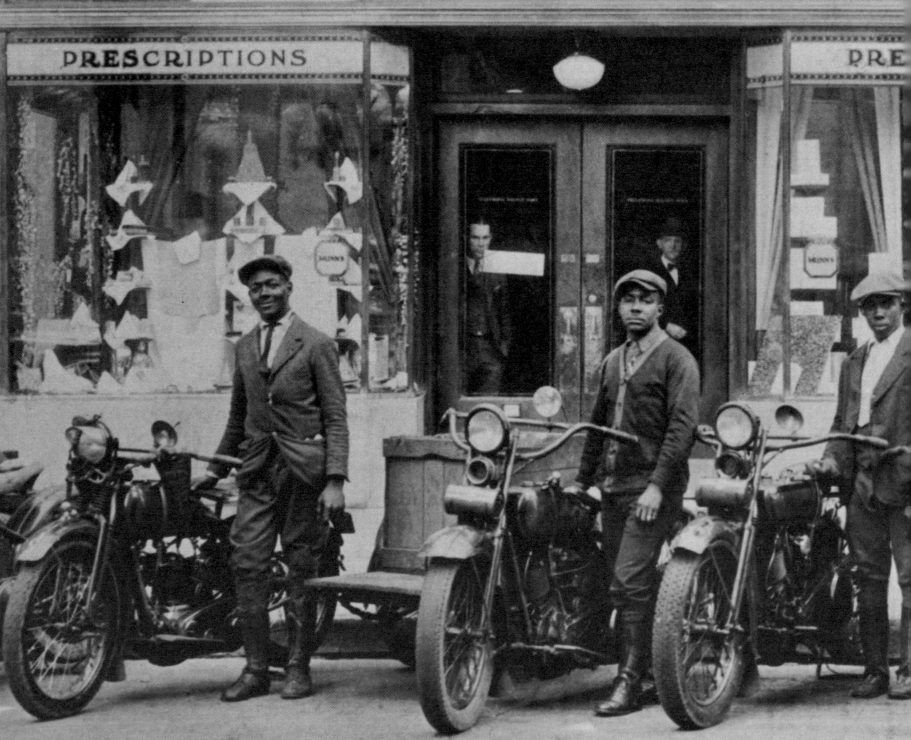

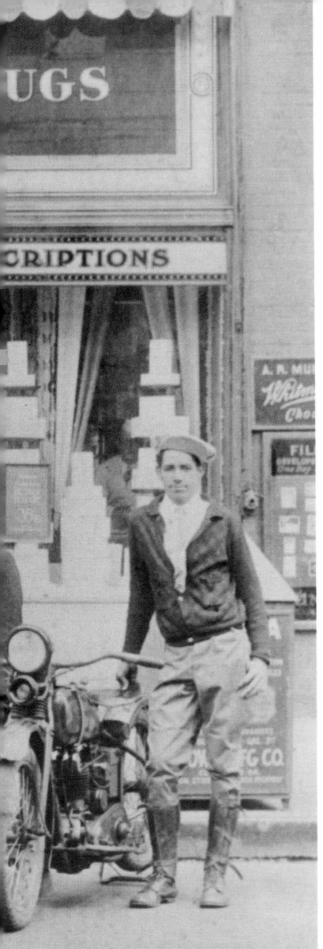

CHAPTER EIGHT

1920-1930

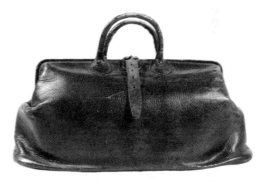

Clean and sterile laboratories were the exceptions when virology emerged as a separate discipline in the 1920s. Thomas G. Rivers then studying parrot fever at the Hospital of Rockefeller Institute, complained bitterly about his unsanitary laboratory to Rufus Cole, the hospital's first director. On March 6, 1930, Cole wrote to his successor, Simon Flexner: ''...Rivers came to me yesterday a little disturbed about the working facilities...Three of the women...have come down with...psittacosis...

''I wish...he might have better facilities than are afforded by the dark room in which they are working. Should not men working on easily transmissible diseases such as yellow fever and psittacosis, have large light rooms in which every precaution to avoid infection can be taken?...''

In addition to pioneer efforts in virology, the 1920s produced remarkable medical discoveries, such as insulin by Frederick Banting and Charles Best. Of particular significance was the growing awareness of dietary insufficiencies and vitamins as a direct cause of disease, as for example of rickets and pernicious anemia.

With the expansion and refinement of medical knowledge and the increasing urban population, physicians were no longer able to deal with all aspects of medicine and the influx of patients. Thus, began a pattern of specialization that characterizes much of contemporary medicine.

Left: Drugstore Deliverymen. Photograph, c. 1920. [A.H.S.] Munn's drugstore, in Atlanta, used a fleet of motorcycles to deliver prescriptions. *Above:* Doctor's Bag. Leather, c. 1920. Photograph, 20th century. [H.M.M.]

1920: 106,446,000 inhabitants; 51.2% urban, 48.8% rural
19th Amendment (women's suffrage) ratified
Warren G. Harding elected President
1920-27: Sacco-Vanzetti, a worldwide cause
1921: Veterans Bureau created
First Immigration Quota Law passed
1922-29: Business boom
1922: Radios in some three million homes
1923: Harding died; Calvin Coolidge, President
Leopold-Loeb murder trial
1925: John T. Scopes found guilty of teaching evolution

1920

1920: Public health nursing was engaged in by some 4,000 organizations employing approximately 11,000 nurses.

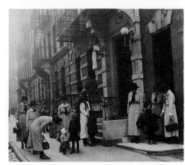

The Visiting Nurse Service of New York

1920: Surgery on the mitral valve of the heart was performed by Elliott C. Cutler of Cleveland.

1921: Insulin was isolated by two Canadians at the University of Western Ontario, Frederick Banting (1891-1941), and Charles H. Best (1899-1978). They isolated the hormone from extracts of pancreas, and demonstrated how injections could replace the natural secretions deficient in diabetics. Until their discovery, only the mildest forms of diabetes could be controlled by strict diets. In 1922, insulin was administered for the first time to a patient, a 14-year-old boy weighing 65 pounds. In the same year, Eli Lilly and Company undertook commercial production of insulin. In 1923, Banting shared the Nobel Prize in physiology and medicine with his director, J. J. R. Macleod.

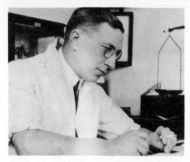

Dr. Frederick Banting

1921: Experimenting with rats suffering from rickets, Paul G. Shipley and Edwards A. Park at Johns Hopkins discovered that sunlight prevented the disease. (The ultraviolet irradiation forms Vitamin D in the skin.)

1921: A new method for taking x-rays of the kidneys was developed by Earl D. Osborne and Leonard G. Rowntree at the Mayo Clinic. Discovering that sodium iodide is opaque to x-rays and that it is rapidly concentrated in the kidneys after injection into a vein, the Mayo collaborators developed a new kind of contrast radiography.

1922: Vitamin D, contained in cod liver oil, was discovered by Elmer V. McCollum and his associates at Johns Hopkins. It was soon recognized as a dietary factor essential for solid bones in children, and as a cure for rickets or rachitis, which causes bow legs, knock knees and deformities of the chest and pelvis.

1922: The Harvard School of Public Health was founded.

1922: The U.S. Public Health Service opened an Office of Cancer Investigation, with a laboratory for cancer research at Harvard.

1922: Walter E. Dandy (1886-1946), a student of Harvey Cushing, was appointed chief of the neurological surgery service at Johns Hopkins. He introduced a new method for the diagnosis and localization of brain tumors, and originated new instruments and operations for hydrocephalus, neuralgias, and aneurysms of the arteries at the base of the brain. His contributions earned him an international reputation.

1922: The existence of Vitamin E was recognized.

1922: The American Society of Clinical Pathologists was founded.

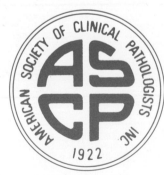

Seal of the American Society of Clinical Pathologists

1923: Another breakthrough in radiology was the development of the Graham test—the use of a phenolphthalein compound to make the gall bladder visible—by Evarts Graham and Warren H. Cole at Washington University, St. Louis. The x-ray method for diagnosing stones and diseases of the gall bladder came into general use.

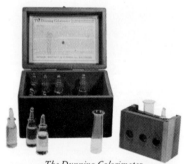

The Dunning Colorimeter, A System for Urinanalysis

1924: The Association of Parasitologists was founded.

1924: The American Protestant Hospital Association was formed.

1925: The parathyroid hormone, parathormone, was isolated and named by James Bertram Collip at the University of Alberta.

1925: Harvey Cushing won the Pulitzer Prize in biography for his *Life of William Osler.*

1927: Charles Lindbergh flew first New York-Paris non-stop flight
The Jazz Singer introduced talking movies

1928: Herbert Hoover elected President
Kellogg-Briand Pact "outlawed" war

1929: Federal Farm Bureau established
Richard E. Byrd flew over the South Pole
Stock Market crash; Great Depression began

1930: Veterans Administration created
123,077,000 inhabitants; 56.2% urban, 43.8 rural

1930

1926: Viruses were distinguished from bacteria in an influential paper presented to the Society of American Bacteriologists by Thomas G. Rivers (1888-1962). Virology was established as a separate discipline, and Rivers' *Filterable Viruses,* the first American textbook devoted to virus diseases, was published in 1928.

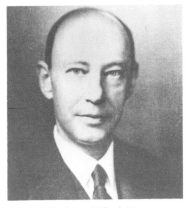

Dr. George Richards Minot

1926: Pernicious anemia, previously a fatal disease, was successfully treated by George Richards Minot (1885-1950), who recognized its cause as dietary deficiency, and prescribed the consumption of liver. The therapeutic substance contained in liver was eventually known as Vitamin B_{12}. Minot was awarded the Nobel Prize in 1934.

1926: Professor John J. Abel of Johns Hopkins Medical School isolated pure crystalline insulin and proved it was a protein.

1926: The first reported case in the United States of histoplasmosis, a lung disease resembling tuberculosis, was described by Cecil J. Watson and W. A. Riley of the University of Minnesota. The microorganism, Histoplasma capsulatum, had been discovered in 1906 in Panama by another American, Samuel Taylor Darling.

1927: Charles Mayo first successfully removed a pheochromocytoma, a functioning adrenal tumor.

1927: An adrenal cortical extract was made by F. A. Hartman and his associates at the University of Buffalo. In 1930 Hartman improved the extract, and yet another was made by W. W. Swingle and J. J. Pfiffner at Princeton. These discoveries made the treatment of Addison's disease (adrenal insufficiency) possible.

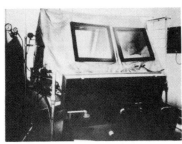

An Oxygen Tent Made by the Oxygen Equipment Manufacturing Corp., of New York

1927: New York Hospital and the Cornell Medical College became affiliated. The new buildings opened in 1932.

1928: The iron lung was invented by Philip Drinker and Louis A. Shaw to facilitate the breathing of polio victims. It was used clinically for the first time in 1929.

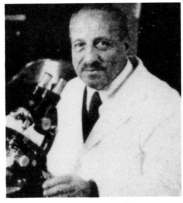

Dr. George Papanicolaou

1928: Diagnosis of uterine cancer was advanced by George Papanicolaou (1883-1962), whose study of cast-off vaginal cells led him to identify malignant cells among the normal. The Pap test was named for its Greek-American developer.

1928: Columbia-Presbyterian Medical Center opened in New York. Although a formal agreement between Columbia University and Presbyterian Hospital was signed in 1911, the war and slow construction had delayed the opening. The College of Physicians and Surgeons was included in the complex.

1928: By international agreement, the roentgen was established as the unit for measurement of x-ray dosage.

1929: Dr. Edward A. Doisy of St. Louis isolated an estrogenic hormone in pure crystalline form. It was considered a breakthrough in hormone research.

1929: The Institute of the History of Medicine was established at Johns Hopkins.

1930: Duke University Hospital and Medical School opened.

1930: The National Institute of Health was established. It grew out of the work of the Hygienic Laboratory of the U.S. Public Health Service, and set the stage for the role of the federal government in medical research.

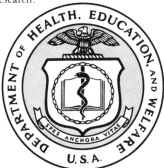

Seal of The National Institute of Health

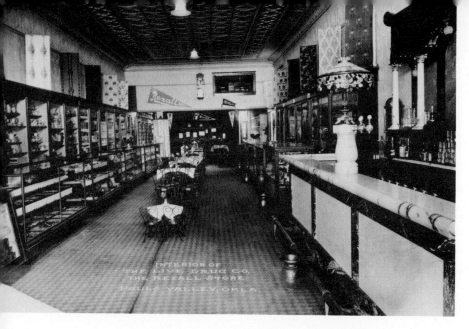

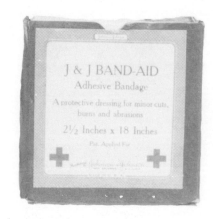

Above: The Live Drug Co., Pauls Valley, Oklahoma. Photograph, early 20th century. [L.C.] As retail pharmacy chains proliferated, the soda fountain, a fixture in most drugstores, became a familiar part of our culture. *Above right:* J & J Band-Aid Adhesive Bandage. Package, 20th century. [J.J.] Introduced in 1920, the Band-Aid Adhesive Bandage was one of the most successful pharmaceutical products of the period. *Below left:* Early Cardiac Clinic. Photograph, 1926. [N.L.M.] In the 1920s, the practice of medicine was fast becoming specialized, and medical institutions reflected the change. Shown is Bellevue Hospital's first cardiac clinic, established in New York in 1925. *Below right:* Black Dentists in New York. Photograph, 1926. [L.C.] The availability and quality of medical and dental education continued to expand in the 1920s, as did the contributions of blacks who were gaining further access to the system.

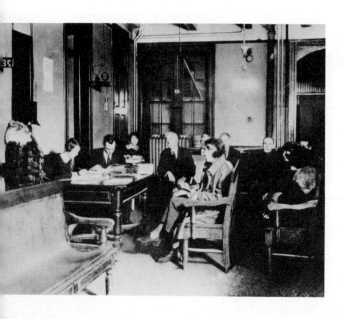

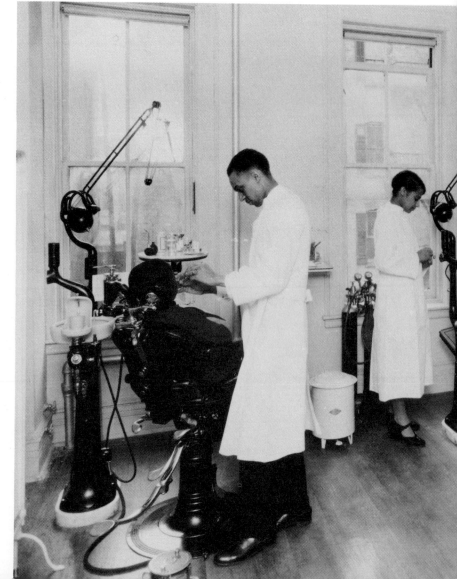

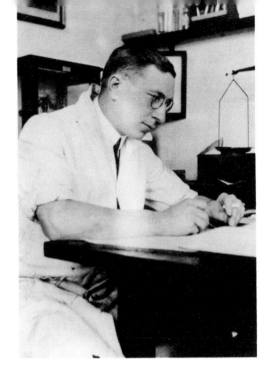

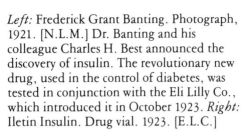

Left: Frederick Grant Banting. Photograph, 1921. [N.L.M.] Dr. Banting and his colleague Charles H. Best announced the discovery of insulin. The revolutionary new drug, used in the control of diabetes, was tested in conjunction with the Eli Lilly Co., which introduced it in October 1923. *Right:* Iletin Insulin. Drug vial. 1923. [E.L.C.]

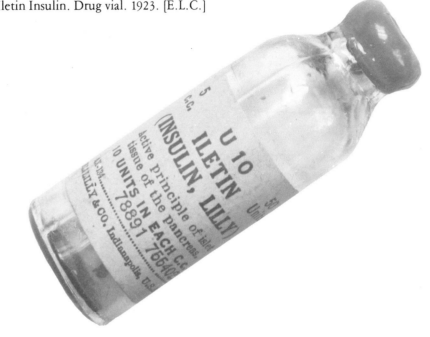

Below: Eli Lilly Research Staff. Photograph, c. 1915. [E.L.C.]

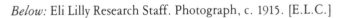

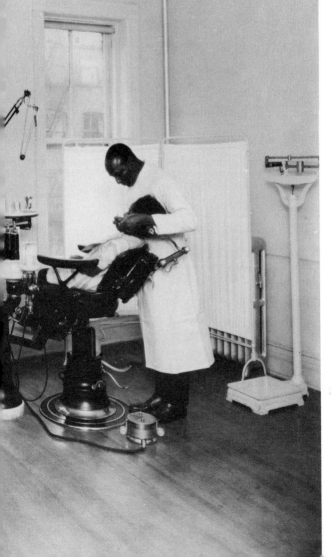

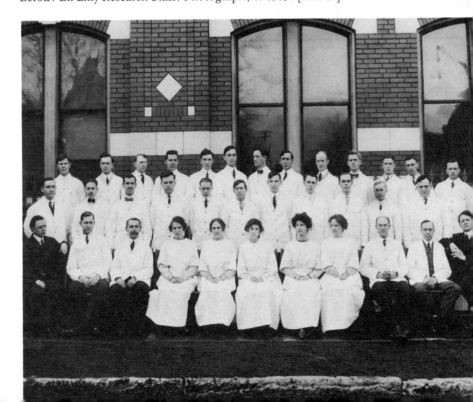

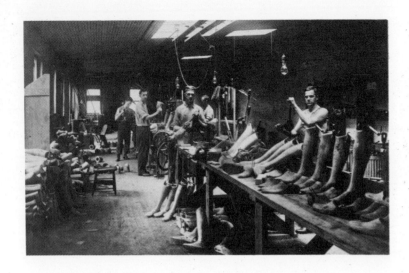

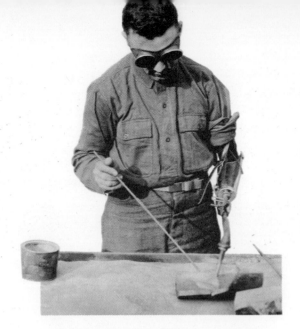

Above: Rehabilitation Training. Photograph, c. 1920. [L.C.] A veteran is seen learning to use an artificial hand. *Left:* J.E. Hanger Shop. Photograph, c. 1916. [L.C.] Artificial limbs for wounded servicemen were custom manufactured in this Washington, D.C. shop. *Below:* Cripples Set for Race, Photograph, c. 1920. [L.C.] Amputees on crutches were encouraged to compete in races as part of their rehabilitation.

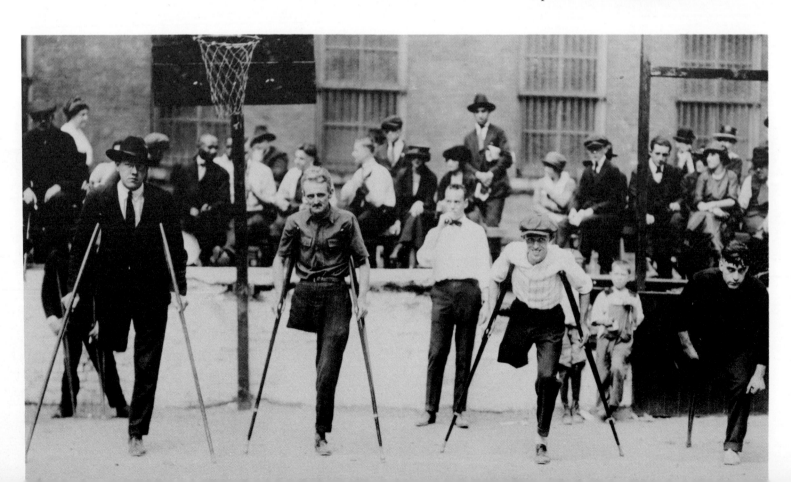

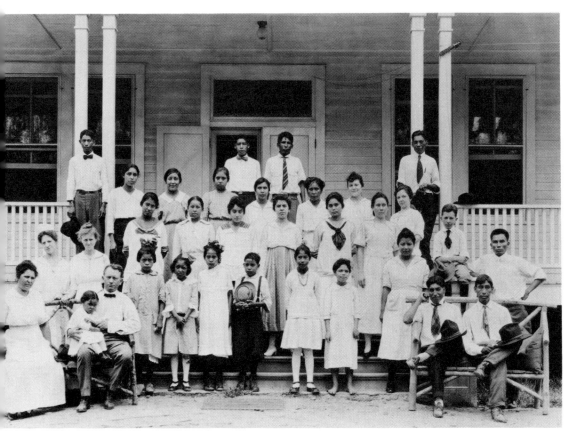

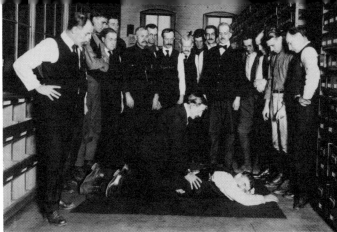

Above: Carter Hospital. Photograph, c. 1920. [L.C.] In the 1920s, many Native Americans were confined to reservations in the West and Southwest. This Oklahoma hospital clinic served Anglos and Native Americans. *Above right:* Emergency Resuscitation Demonstration. Photograph, c. 1922. [L.C.] Government office workers in Washington, D.C. were shown the technique of artificial respiration, a crucial part of first aid education. *Right:* TB Health Stamp. Photograph, 1924. [M.H.S.] The 1920s saw an increase in publicity and fund-raising events for health causes. This tableau, presented in Minnesota in 1924, was part of a Christmas Seal sale for the benefit of the National Tuberculosis Foundation.

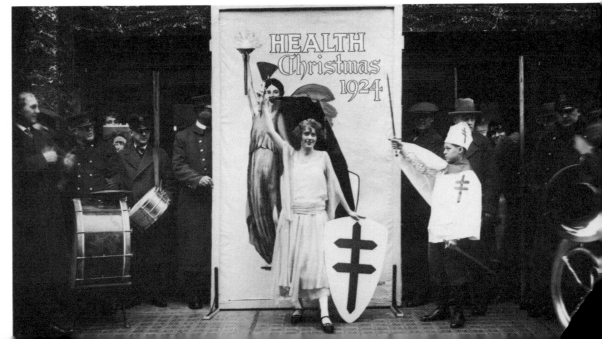

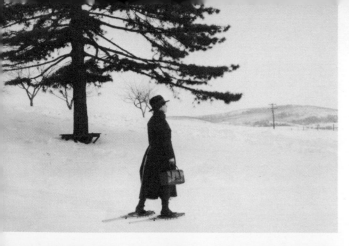

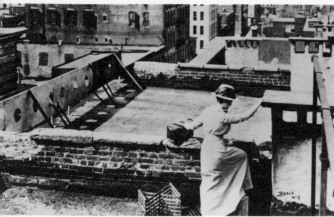

Left: Rural Health Nurse on Snowshoes. Photograph, 1925. [M.27.] Photographed by Lewis Hine in the Ramapo Mountains of New Jersey. *Below left:* A Member of the Visiting Nurse Service of New York. Photograph, c. 1920. [V.N.S.N.Y.] She is seen clambering over a tenement roof to reach her patient-client. *Right:* Providing Day Care. Photograph, 1926. [V.N.S.N.Y.] Five nurses posed with five sets of twins then in their care. *Bottom:* Graduation Class. Photograph, early 20th century. [A.H.S.] The first graduating class of nurses at Atlanta's Wesley Memorial Hospital posed for this portrait.

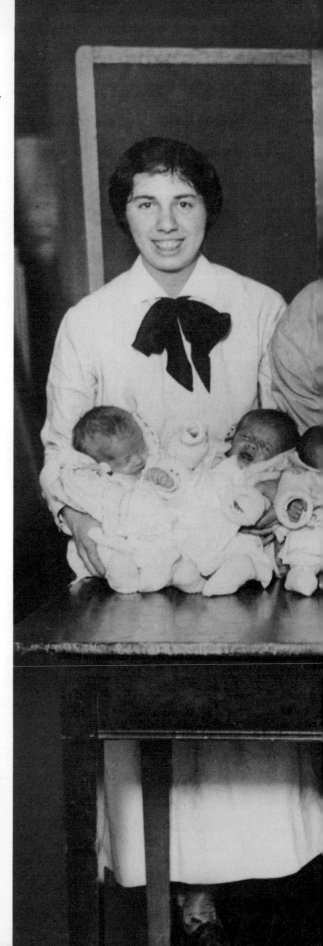

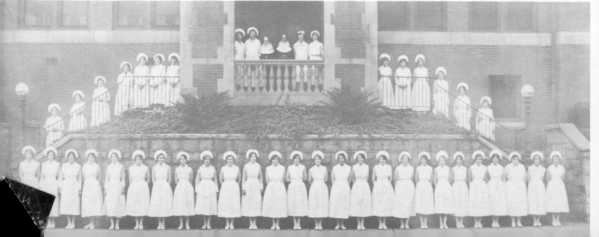

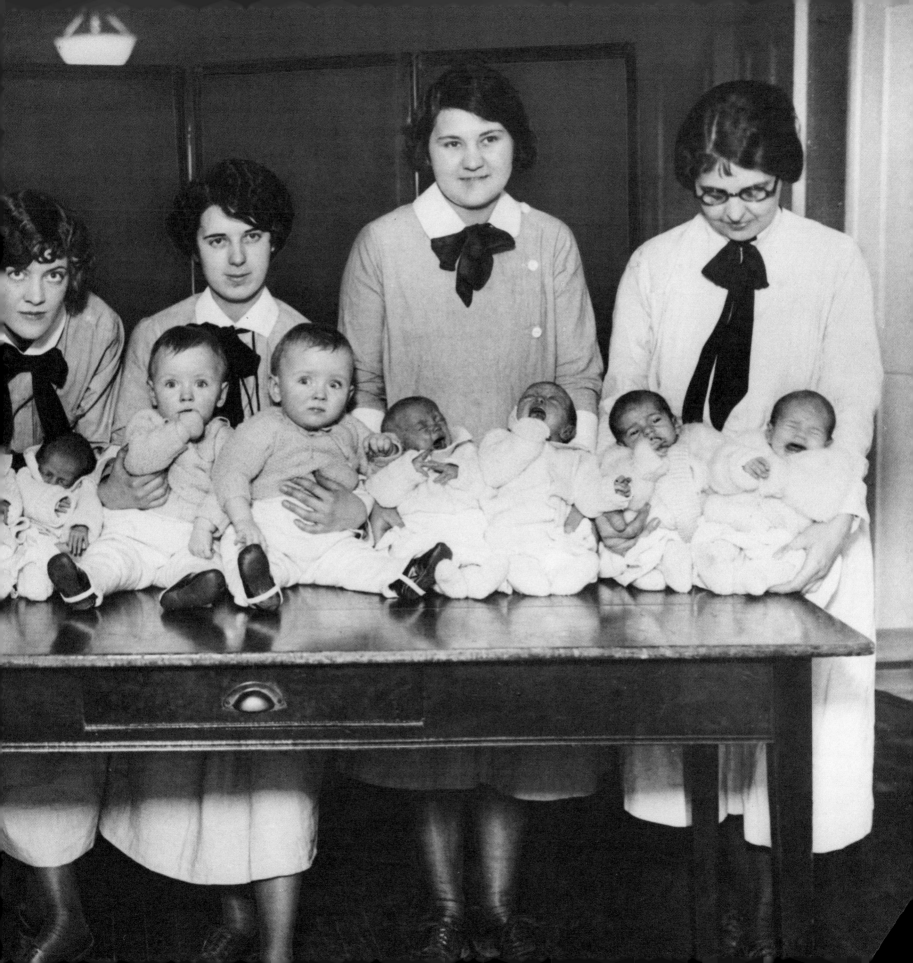

Acknowledgments and Bibliography

Acknowledgments

The editors are immensely grateful to numbers of individuals for sharing their expertise with us and granting permission to reproduce material from their collections and institutions.

In the caption for each basic illustration herein there appears a bracketed letter/ number code indicating the source of the image. The key to those designations is as follows:

AHS — Atlanta Historical Society
AMA — American Medical Association
APA — American Pharmaceutical Association
APS — American Philosophical Society
BM — Bristol-Myers Company
CHM — Cooper-Hewitt Museum Library Picture Collection, Kubler Collection, Smithsonian Institution
CHS — Chicago Historical Society
DOA — Department of the Army
ELC — Eli Lilly and Company
EMH — Ephraim McDowell House
ERS — E.R. Squibb & Sons, Inc.
FLI — Frederic Lewis, Inc.
HMM — Heustis Medical Museum, University of South Alabama
HMPS — Historic Mobile Preservation Society
HMS — Hartford Medical Society
JJ — Johnson and Johnson
LC — The Library of Congress
LCP — The Library Company of Philadelphia
MCNY — The Museum of the City of New York
MGH — Massachusetts General Hospital
MHS — Minnesota Historical Society
MJC — Mead Johnson & Company
NA — National Archives, General Services Administration
NLM — National Library of Medicine
NMHT — National Museum of History and Technology, Smithsonian Institution
NYAM — New York Academy of Medicine
NYCDH — New York City Department of Health
NYPL/PC — New York Public Library Picture Collection
PC — Private Collection
PCP — Philadelphia College of Pharmacy
PCPS — Philadelphia College of Physicians & Surgeons
PH — Pennsylvania Hospital
SHSW — State Historical Society of Wisconsin
SKC — SmithKline Corporation
SPUW — School of Pharmacy, University of Wisconsin

TL — Baxter Travenol Laboratories, Inc.
US — University of the South
USA — University of South Alabama Photographic Archives, Erik Overbey/Mobile Public Library Collection
USNA — U.S. Naval Academy Museum
VFHS — Valley Forge Historical Society
VNSNY — Visiting Nurse Service of New York
WLC — Warner-Lambert Company

Miscellaneous Codes:

M1: Connecticut Valley Historical Museum, Springfield, MA
M2: Musée des Arts Décoratifs, The Louvre, Paris
M3: Archives Nationales: Section Outre-mer, Paris
M4: The Mount Sinai Hospital
M5: The Royal College of Surgeons of England
M6: Ohio Historical Society
M7: George M. Cushing Photography
M8: Temple University School of Dentistry
M9: Coca Cola Company
M10: St. Louis Metropolitan Medical Society
M11: The Bettmann Archive
M12: The Johns Hopkins University School of Medicine
M13: Historic Westville Restoration, Lumpkin, Georgia
M14: The Johns Hopkins University Press
M15: Bancroft Library, University of California, Berkeley
M16: National Gallery of Art
M17: Brown Brothers
M18: Culver Pictures, Inc.
M19: Thomas Jefferson University
M20: Presbyterian Hospital, New York City
M21: The Upjohn Company
M22: Lane County Museum, Eugene, Oregon
M23: Clark University Archives
M24: Moorland-Spingarn Research Center, Washington, D.C.
M25: Norwich-Eaton Pharmaceuticals
M26: Western Reserve Historical Society
M27: George Eastman House

In addition, we gratefully acknowledge use of the illustrations in the eight time lines as follows:
Chapter One (left to right): 1-4: PC; 5: PCPS; 6: PC; 7: HMS
Chapter Two: 1: NLM; 2: LCP; 3: NLM; 4: PC; 5,6: APS; 7: LC
Chapter Three: 1: NYAM; 2: NLM; 3: PH; 4: NLM; 5: AMA; 6: HMM; 7: CHM; 8: LC

Chapter Four: 1,2: NLM; 3: LC; 4: NLM; 5: JJ; 6: NYAM; 7,8: NLM; 9: ELC; 10: WLC
Chapter Five: 1: M21; 2: PCPS; 3: JJ; 4,5: NLM; 6: LC
Chapter Six: 1: NLM; 2-4: LC; 7: M18
Chapter Seven: 1: US; 2: LC; 3: JJ; 4: NLM; 5: MHS; 6-8: LC
Chapter Eight: 1: VNSNY; 2: NLM; 3,4: NYAM; 5: NLM; 6,7: NYAM

Limited space precludes our being able to list all those who have helped us, but we particularly wish to thank the following:

Gilbert F. Martin at the American Medical Association; Dr. Eugene Craig at the Atlanta Historical Society; Helen Davidson at Eli Lilly and Company; Dr. Samuel Eichold and Terry Anderson at the Heustis Medical Museum at the University of South Alabama; Sidney Adair Smith at the Historic Mobile Preservation Society; Myrna Williamson at the Historical Society of Wisconsin; Peggy Pearse and Tom Murphy at Johnson & Johnson; Bonnie Wilson at the Minnesota Historic Society; Elizabeth Moyer and Gretchen Worden at the Mütter Museum of the Philadelphia College of Physicians and Surgeons; Lucinda Keister and Astrid Ottey at the National Library of Medicine; Sallie Morgenstern and Miriam Mandelbaum at the New York Academy of Medicine; Doris P. Shalley at SmithKline Corporation; Julian Aurelius at Squibb; Sherry S. Kaplan at Baxter Travenol Laboratories, Inc.; Mrs. Arnold Mignery at the University of the South; Joan Tabb at the Visiting Nurse Service of New York; Thorn Kuhl at Warner-Lambert Company.

Finally, our deep appreciation to George B. Griffenhagen of the American Pharmaceutical Association, and Dr. William D. Sharpe, who provided valuable counsel in addition to their respective Foreword and Introduction.

Carter Smith

A Selected Bibliography

Bennion, Elizabeth. *Antique Medical Instruments.* Berkeley and Los Angeles: University of California Press, 1979.

Bettman, Otto C. *A Pictorial History of Medicine.* Springfield, Ill.: Charles C. Thomas, 1956.

Bordley, James III and McGehee, Harvey A. *Two Centuries of American Medicine, 1776-1976.* Philadelphia: W.B. Saunders Co. 1976.

DePauw, Linda Grant and Hunt, Conover. *Remember the Ladies.* New York: Viking Press, 1976.

Garrison, Fielding H. *History of Medicine.* Philadelphia: W.B. Saunders, 1929.

Griffenhagen, George B. *Drug Supplies in the American Revolution.* Washington, D.C.: Smithsonian Institution, 1961.

Holbrook, Stewart H. *The Golden Age of Quackery.* New York: Macmillan and Co., 1959.

Hurd-Mead, K.C. *A History of Women in Medicine.* 1938. Reprint. Boston: Milford House, 1973.

Kahn, E.J., Jr. *All in a Century.* Indianapolis: Eli Lilly and Co., 1976.

Kremers, E. and Urdang, G. *History of Pharmacy.* Rev. ed. Philadelphia: J.B. Lippincott Co., 1976.

Lee, Russel V.; Eimerl, Sarel and the Editors of Time-Life Books. *The Physician.* New York: Time-Life Books, 1968.

Lyons, Albert S. and Petrucelli, R. Joseph. *Medicine, an Illustrated History.* New York: Harry N. Abrams, 1978.

Marion, John Francis. *The Fine Old House.* Philadelphia: SmithKline Corp., 1980.

_____. *Philadelphia Medica.* Harrisburg: SmithKline Corp., 1975.

Modell, Walter; Lansing, Alfred and the Editors of Life. *Drugs.* New York: Time, Inc., 1967.

Rush, Benjamin. *The Autobiography of Benjamin Rush.* Edited by George W. Corner. Princeton: Princeton University Press, 1948.

Shryock, Richard H. *Medicine and Society in America, 1660-1860.* New York: New York University Press, 1960.

Sigerist, Henry E. *The Great Doctors: A Biographical History of Medicine.* Translated by Eder and Cedar Paul. Garden City, N.Y.: Doubleday & Co., Anchor Books, 1958.

Thorwald, Jurgen. *The Century of a Surgeon.* New York: Pantheon Books, 1956.

Vogel, Virgil J. *American Indian Medicine.* Norman: University of Oklahoma Press, 1970.

Weinberger, Bernhard Wolf. *An Introduction to the History of Dentistry.* St. Louis: C.V. Mosby Co., 1948.

Werner, D. *History of the Red Cross.* London: Cassell & Co., 1941.

Index

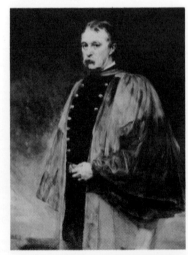

Dr. John Shaw Billings. As the first director of the National Library of Medicine (1865-1895), General Billings was principally responsible for building that archive into the world's foremost collection of biomedical literature.